Also by Darcey Steinke

FICTION

Sister Golden Hair
Milk
Jesus Saves
Suicide Blonde
Up Through the Water

NONFICTION

Easter Everywhere

Flash Count Diary

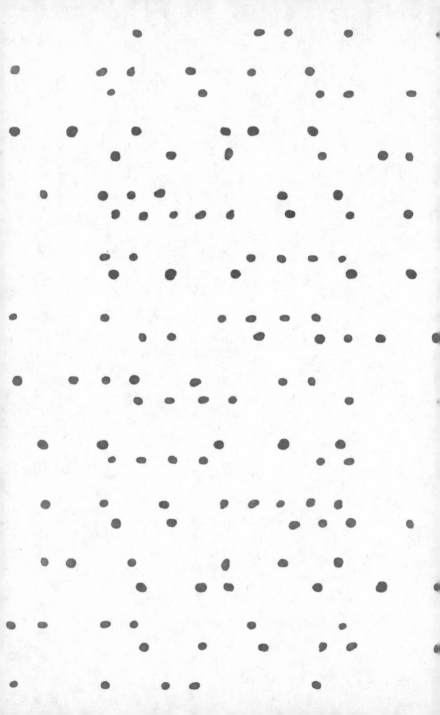

Flash Count Diary

Menopause

and the

Vindication

of Natural Life

Darcey Steinke

Sarah Crichton Books   Farrar, Straus and Giroux • New York

Sarah Crichton Books
Farrar, Straus and Giroux
120 Broadway, New York 10271

Library of Congress Cataloging-in-Publication Data
Names: Steinke, Darcey, author.
Title: Flash count diary : menopause and the vindication of natural life /
    Darcey Steinke.
Description: First Edition. | New York : Sarah Crichton Books / Farrar,
    Straus and Giroux, [2019] | Includes bibliographical references.
Identifiers: LCCN 2018046534 | ISBN 9780374156114 (hardcover)
Subjects: LCSH: Women—Psychology. | Menopause. | Sexism.
Classification: LCC HQ1206 .S734 2019 | DDC 155.3/33—dc23
LC record available at https://lccn.loc.gov/2018046534

Designed by Abby Kagan

Our books may be purchased in bulk for promotional, educational,
or business use. Please contact your local bookseller or the Macmillan
Corporate and Premium Sales Department at 1-800-221-7945, extension
5442, or by e-mail at MacmillanSpecialMarkets@macmillan.com.

www.fsgbooks.com
www.twitter.com/fsgbooks • www.facebook.com/fsgbooks

10   9   8   7   6   5   4   3   2   1

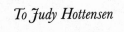

To Judy Hottensen

Our bodies too are always and endlessly changing;
what we have been today, we shall not be tomorrow.
—OVID

The body is not a thing but a situation.
—SIMONE DE BEAUVOIR

If I had to choose between the two phases of life,
I am truly not sure on which my choice would fall.
For when one leaves erotic experience in the narrower
sense, one is at the same time leaving a cul-de-sac,
however marvelous it may be, where there is only
room for two abreast, and one now continues, upon a
vast expanse—the expanse of which childhood too
was a part and which for only a while we were bound
to forget.
—LOU ANDREAS-SALOMÉ

Something tender, secret, and painful draws out the
intimacy which keeps vigil in us, extending its
glimmer into that animal darkness.
—GEORGES BATAILLE

Then animals long believed gone crept down
From trees. We took stock of one another.
—TRACY K. SMITH

Contents

1. Night on Fire   3
2. Free Lolita   22
3. The Animals   37
4. Mind at the End of Its Tether   53
5. Demigirl in Kemmering   78
6. Lessons in Demonology   95
7. The Old Monkey   114
8. Nocturnal Hunter   144
9. Hole in My Heart   162
10. The Whale Wins   179
11. Home Waters   206

A Note About the Whales   219
Notes   221
Acknowledgments   227

Flash Count Diary

1 ● Night on Fire

2:11 a.m.: I wake, heart thwacking, as heat flows up from my stomach, courses behind my face, and radiates out through the top of my head. I watch a lamp with a pink shade drift out of my neighbor's window and hover over my darkened backyard.

An hour later I wake again, this time within the aura before the flash. No matter my mood, each aura brings a surreal déjà vu feeling, the "thorn in the flesh" that Saint Paul talked about: everything is stilled, everything is wrong. It's as if a shard of a different and darker reality has been thrust into my current one.

Auras are less universal than heat, though many in the diverse group of women I interviewed reported having them.

"About a minute before the flash comes I get the worst feeling," one woman told me. Another described the eerie quiet just before the feeling of thick unease: "I get very calm, then a sensation comes that scares the heck out of me." Another experiences a free fall: "I feel like I'm going down in an elevator, my stomach drops, flash of nausea, a weird weak feeling, then the heat."

I throw off my covers and feel, in the first pocket of spooky quiet, that flames are burning from my inner organs up into my muscles toward the skin. I'd run away, but how does one flee one's own body? Each hair is a thin electric coil heating up my head.

I know what's going to happen and I know that it's going to be bizarre. I leap up and go into the kitchen, run myself a glass of cold water, gulp it down. I jerk a bag of corn out of the freezer and press it against my chest and stare out the window. The leaves in the yard blow one way and then the other. I go back to bed, but the heat coming off my husband's body is dangerous. I go into my daughter's empty room and lie in her bed surrounded by posters for DIY bands and photos of her high school girlfriends. Her thick comforter triggers another flash. First comes the stillness, the "sinister feeling" one woman described. I feel outside continuous conventional reality, trapped inside the flesh-and-blood corporeality of my body. Saint Paul, who may have had epilepsy, called his auras "an intimation of heaven." Not the cliché fluffy-cloud angelic sphere but a feeling of the next life in all its raw, brutal grandeur. I yank up the window. Heat sweeps through me like a tiny weather front. I know my parcel of the earth is spinning closer to the sun and the air is heating up. Even a few degrees' rise, when my windows are open, can trigger a flash.

Much like my sense of smell was magnified when I was pregnant, my body is now sensitive to the smallest calibrations of heat. When food is placed in front of me at a restaurant, most recently a plate of scrambled eggs, first my belly and then my face burn. Entering a room, I won't at first know it's sealed, but as I talk to a student in my office or teach in my classroom, the sense of entrapment grows. I'll glance at the window, the door, panicking as one after another, body, room, building, is locked down tight. As the fire bowls along my nerves, I long to escape my body, to shoot up through my own skin, the ceiling, and bust into the atmosphere itself.

When I wake next, there is smoky light at the window and the heat in my limbs is already subsiding. I shift. My husband asks what's wrong. *It's happening again*, I say, jolting up, running the tap in the kitchen, drinking down the cold water. I go back to the couch, and though the windows are open, they face a brick wall. I feel trapped in the narrow room, squeezed.

My Flash Count Diary, a mottled black-and-white composition book, lies on the coffee table. Nine flashes today, not counting this current run. First, over coffee this morning, I felt my heart compress and then heat launch out horizontally into my arms and down into my hands. Later, while teaching, talking about how blankness as an interior state for a fictional character has to be created, just like anger or desire, I felt a sudden pang of misery followed by a smoldering sensation in my back. After class, out for a drink with a friend, listening to her talk about her husband's hallucinations, I felt heat radiate from my stomach up into my chest, neck, rolling up like steam behind my face. Once home, I flashed while washing dishes and changing the kitty litter. And finally, just before bed, I had the sensation that my nightgown was affixed to my body with hot glue.

Back in my bedroom, I am trying again to sleep. It's almost daylight as I make a pallet out of blankets on the floor next to our bed. I want to be near my husband. I lie, one leg out of the blanket, calf pressed against the cold wood. I must always be a little cooler than is comfortable in order not to flash.

I have found flashes to be desperate, uncomfortable, sometimes even sublime, but never funny. On TV and in film, if they are shown at all, hot flashes are comedic bits akin to a man slipping on a banana peel. As a child, I remember watching Edith Bunker on *All in the Family* redden, fan herself, get discombobulated, and dash into the kitchen as the laugh track roared. Menopause is often filtered through male bafflement and repugnance. In *Mrs. Doubtfire*, Robin Williams catches his fake breasts on fire and, using two pan lids, eventually puts out the flames. He stands disheveled, his chest smoking. "My first day as a woman," he says, "and I am already having hot flashes."

Kitty Forman on *That '70s Show* is menopausal, complaining about the heat and snapping at her family. Her husband, Red, refers to "the horrible thing that has taken over your mother." When Red looks up *menopause* in the encyclopedia, he is repelled. "Good god, I didn't think they'd have pictures."

Jokes about menopause abound.

Q: What is scarier? A puppy or a rational woman in menopause?
A: A puppy, because a rational woman in menopause does not exist.

Q: What is ten times worse than a woman in menopause?
A: Two women in menopause.

Q: Why do women stop bleeding in menopause?
A: They need the blood for their varicose veins.

Women, too, make fun of flashes. On Etsy you can buy buttons that read BEWARE OF TEMPERATURE TANTRUMS and OUT OF ESTROGEN: APPROACH AT YOUR OWN RISK.

Humor can be a way out. A means to exalt and redeem what might otherwise be unbearable. I get that. Humor, as in the work of Samuel Beckett, can show the absurdity of life, of living in a body. "Nothing is funnier than unhappiness," Beckett once said. "It's the most comical thing in the world."

The laughter around hot flashes, though, is not life-affirming. It's thin, strained, and often mean-spirited. Some men are bewildered by the changes in their partners' bodies. They suffer a parallel loss, but their honest grief is too often channeled into misogyny. Many women are fearful that the loss of fertility will take away their femininity. This unexamined shame rushes headlong into self-abasement and produces a brittle humor that is more a symptom of humiliation than actual catharsis.

None of the women I spoke to thought flashes were funny, but all were surprised, as I was, at the severity and isolation of the flash.

—At 3:00 p.m. it hits you like a ton of hot charcoal.
—Hot flashes for me are so severe that I fear I will have a heart attack and die.

—Mine start with . . . fear. It's a quick burst of heat and nerve endings igniting in fear.

—They are like four-minute surprise anxiety attacks. I want to grab at my clothing, find a fan, open the fridge, whatever I can do.

Heat and panic drive many women out of doors for relief. One told me she often finds herself standing in the yard, flapping her pajamas in the middle of the night. Another puts on a sundress and stands barefoot in her freezing garage, surrounded by the tools on her husband's workbench.

I often grab stuff out of my freezer—peas, pita bread, strawberries—and plunk them on my forehead, chest, and stomach. I'll admit that the manic way I run to the fridge, pull out items, throw myself onto the couch, and lie with a slab of frozen ham balanced on my forehead might appear funny. But my flash is much more than a comedic skit. Though no one wants to say it out loud, menopause is about loss; it's about departure—each flash reminds me of my corporeality, my mortality. With every flash, my psyche is pushed to grasp what it does not want to let itself know: that it is not immortal. This is terrifying. It's also a rare opportunity, if faced directly, to come to terms with the limitations of the self.

Looking beyond boilerplate misogyny, I'd argue that the flash has been debased because it's a sort of conduit, a profound crossing to the older stage of life. The sensation I have in the aura before the flash is elevated, possibly even hallucinatory, though that does not diminish its power: I feel I will soon find out knowledge no one else possesses, something to do with the boundary between life and death.

Of the spiritual dimensions of the flash, I find little to nothing in the scientific and self-help literature of menopause. Most of the writing deals with how to get rid of hot flashes, not how to understand them. Premarin, a hormone replacement made out of the urine of pregnant horses, is the most common suggestion. Natural remedies are more humane but vary in effect. Herbalists recommend black cohosh, nettle, soy, rose hip, creams made from wild yam, vitamin E, and vitamin B. One website suggests taking a tablespoon of apple cider vinegar twice a day and another drinking 10 percent of your body weight in water. Belinda Carlisle, the singer from the Go-Go's, recommends putting a magnet in your underpants.

Many online essays urge me to laugh at myself more and complain less. Nobody wants to hear about menopause, even menopausal women themselves. Other female milestones are of more general interest. There is a whole literary genre, the coming-of-age novel, that addresses the move from girlhood to womanhood, and both men and women write about birth as a liminal event. Outside sex, men are never keen on hearing how our bodies feel, but both the onset of fertility/

sexuality and birth are of interest to them in a way that menopause is not.

But what of my feelings—embodied for the first time in a flash—that I am divided, split into soul and body, that there is a *me*, lonely and frantic, who wants out of my corporeal form?

Charles Finney, leader of the First Great Awakening, detailed his religious conversion in language similar to how I and other women describe a flash. In his memoir, he says that his heart seemed to be liquid fire: "My feelings seemed to rise and flow out—like a wave of electricity." Another convert reported that she felt a presence traveling over her: "Suddenly there seemed to be something sweeping into me and inflating my entire being."

Some describe conversion as pleasurable, but for most it's eerie, even frightening. In *Varieties of Religious Experience*, William James collected conversion testimonials: "Suddenly without a moment's warning my whole being seemed roused to the highest state of tension or aliveness, and I was aware, with an intention not easily imagined by those who had never experienced it, that another being or presence was not only in the room, but quite close to me."

In an earlier era, I might have felt the flash as wicked as easily as divine: a witch's spell that sends waves of heat into my body, makes my tongue blaze, gives me the feeling, just under my right elbow, of a strong electrical shock. James, being a psychologist, believed religious conversions were caused by "an underground life," which led a "parasitic existence, buried outside of the primary field of consciousness." During a flash I reside in the liminal; I feel that the membrane between me and another world is worn thin. James felt his scientific explanation of conversion was also compatible with the idea of a higher power: "The notion of a subconscious self certainly ought not at this point in our inquiry be held to exclude all notions of a higher penetration."

Religious conversion, if we believe in it, is an experience of divinity unmediated by doctrine, hymns, or prayers. Those conduits that the transcendentalists thought blocked our relationship with divinity also serve to protect individuals from the full scourging force of the godhead. In conversion that safety filter is blown off its hinges, and believers feel unnerved, nauseated, filled with lava-like heat.

I've been having flashes now for nearly two years. Their onslaught has wiped out the composure and integrity of my old self. "Everyone wants to be the person she was before," Gail Sheehy writes in her book about menopause, *Silent Passage.* But I am no longer my old self, and I can't go backward. Why would I want to take hormone supplements, as Sheehy both advocates doing and did herself to start menstruating again, to dupe my body back into thinking it can still make babies? The feminist Germaine Greer has said that during her brief period on hormones, she didn't like the feeling of going back into the cycle. She felt she had spied another region, one beyond sexual desire and hormonal docility, and wanted to get back there.

There are things I miss about my old self: the ferocity of physical desire, the sense of well-being (aside from the days before my period) that appears to have been in part hormonal, and the fantasy, no matter how ephemeral, that I might have another child. Now I am dinged up, less "moist," as Sheehy so annoyingly points out. But the brokenness that the hot flashes and sleeplessness have wrought feels *real*—a realness that encompasses a wider emotional sweep, a larger sense of the world, and a keener awareness of my own self. Dr. Pauline Maki, of the Center for Research on Women and Gender at the University of Minnesota, told me that one unexpected side effect of hot flashes is greater empathy: "The hot flash comes unbidden. You can't control your body, and this makes women more empathetic to others who are suffering."

The suffragette Elizabeth Cady Stanton, a mother of seven, writes in her memoir that the best part of a woman's life is the back side of fifty, when her energies are not scattered in housework, "when philanthropy takes the place of family selfishness, and when from the depths of poverty and suffering the wail of humanity grows as pathetic to her ears as once was the cry of her own children."

Many women feel during menopause that an old self is dying and, as one woman, an actress and a health coach, told me, "a new creature is trying to get out." Another woman, a young-adult novelist, told me that her flashes begin with her heart hammering so hard and fast that it feels like it's trying to batter its way out of her chest: "I feel like I'm going to burst out of my skin and roar like the Incredible Hulk."

During a recent sleepless night as a flash came on, I got so frustrated that I kicked the stack of books by my bed and squeezed my fists together; then out of my mouth came a deep and guttural roar. "Don't make me angry," Bruce Banner, a.k.a. the Hulk, often warns those around him, knowing that high emotion will raise his pulse and bring on his transformation. Ang Lee's film *Hulk* opens with Banner trying to cure his condition (Banner was blasted with radioactive gamma rays while testing a bomb for the military) with two natural remedies often suggested to menopausal women: herbs and meditation. Later in the film, when his girlfriend asks him what his metamorphosis feels like, he replies, "It's like someone has poured a liter of acid into my brain."

The Hulk was created for Marvel comics by Stan Lee and Jack Kirby in the early sixties, but it's Bill Bixby's and Lou Ferrigno's portrayals of Dr. Banner and the Hulk, respectively, in the seventies television show that most relate to my experience of the change. The show, with its barren-desert

landscapes and makeshift sets, is permeated with alienation and sadness. Banner's melancholy suggests to me that
while the Hulk is make-believe, his burden is real. He
struggles to control his out-of-whack body chemistry and
also "the raging spirit that dwells within him."

YouTube has hundreds of "Hulk Outs," short clips from the
TV show in which Banner changes into the Hulk. Banner is
in a variety of situations: held against his will in a small-town
jail, chasing pickpockets, trapped in a car in a demolition
derby, tied up in a wax museum. The situations are different
but the steps in his mutation are always the same: his face
flushes, his forehead gleams with sweat, and there is an
expression of panic, of his not wanting this to happen.
Before he turns green, his face is open, tentative—an
expression similar to my own when I watched myself flash
in the bathroom mirror, troubled features flooded with
animal longing.

The Hulk, monsterly kin to both Frankenstein's creation and
Mr. Hyde, differs from other superheroes. He goes after bad
guys and saves damsels in distress, but his violence is also chaotic. He'll bust up any room, even his own bedroom. His
rage is inchoate, what with his dead mother, his messed-up
childhood, his chemical imbalance, and his inability to control his own body. The flash is chemical and emotional, en-
compassing past and current frustrations. It is also a means
of self-expression. After years of docility, Banner can reveal

his rage. Greer writes in her book *The Change* that some of our negative feelings about menopause are "the result of our intolerance for the expression of female anger." In menopause women come up, as never before, against their own mentality.

The change for decades has been a euphemism for menopause, whispered behind the backs of aging women: *She's going through the change.* It sounds sinister and surreal but is actually accurate. Like the Hulk, I don't have symptoms or a condition; I am in the midst of a rupture, a metamorphosis, an all-encompassing and violent *change*.

I watch Bixby's chest bloat, the buttons fly off his plaid shirt, his green skin expand like the stem of a gigantic plant. Seams split, his belt pops, even the leather of his boots explodes. He is out of control but also free. And while he may break down a few doors, he also acts with an inner integrity. "The woman who lashes out at menopause," Greer writes, "has found the breach in her self-discipline through which she may be able, finally, to escape to liberty."

Freedom is on the horizon—freedom from child care and domestic duties, from trying to be beautiful, from the leering male gaze, from derailing sexual desires. First, however, my body must evolve. As a woman, I should be used to the seismic changes of flesh and blood. During puberty my skin got greasy, my breasts popped out, and I started, to my

astonishment, growing black hairs under my arms and between my legs. During the last month of my pregnancy, the
creature inside me often jammed a toe into my stomach
and dragged that toe across the curved plane of my protruding belly. In both puberty and pregnancy, I was often mysti-
fied, but there were also solid gains to look forward to—a
grown-up female body, sex, a baby.

The bodily changes the flash forewarns—vaginal entropy,
wrinkles, bones crumbling with osteoporosis—are less hopeful, even grim. "So we die before our own eyes," Sarah Orne
Jewett wrote in 1898. "We see some chapters of our lives come
to their natural end." The Bulgarian-French philosopher
Julia Kristeva locates horror, which she calls the abject, in the
moment we are reminded we are living in a body. "Abjection
is above all ambiguity. Because, while releasing a hold, it does
not actually cut off the subject from what threatens it—on the
contrary, abjection acknowledges it to be a perpetual danger." What frightens me most—decay, death—*is me.*

◎ ◎ ◎

It would be hard to find a structure more abject than the Port
Authority Bus Terminal in New York City. It reminds me of
what purgatory might look like: smeared glass, grubby tile,
exhausted souls slumped on plastic chairs and waiting on line.
I've just taught my class at Columbia, and I'm going back up
to our little cottage in Sullivan County to help my husband

close down the place for the winter. The bus is full of slack-faced men in ill-fitting suits and women in polyester floral dresses. Walking down the bus's center aisle, I pass a large lady in a pink tracksuit and a bald man wearing Elvis sunglasses. I find a window seat near the back. The elderly man beside me is talking on his cell phone about his appointment in the city. He got mixed signals from his doctor about whether he is going to live or die.

For now the bus door is open, but once it closes I'll be sealed in, and though I have on three removable layers, not counting my sports bra, I know I am bound to flash.

I knew so much more going into both menstruation and pregnancy than I did going into menopause. Part of this is because secrecy, shame, and fear still stigmatize the change. But the other part is that so little is known for certain about menopause and the science of hot flashes. Because there are few good animal models—the only creatures that go through menopause are human women, female killer whales, narwhals, and short-finned pilot and beluga whales—most of what we know about how the body works in menopause is speculation. Studies have found that flashes are associated with decreased levels of hormones and that these decreases confuse the vasomotor system.

The vasomotor system includes the brain's brain, the hypothalamus, as well as the stomach, the central nervous system, internal organs, the spinal cord, and skin. Cilia and fibers in all these systems send information to the hypothalamus about our body temperature. Think of the hypothalamus as the main control center of the New York City subway system and of the outer vasomotor system as the various stations and miles of track. Hormones make this system run smoothly. During our reproductive years, our brains grow addicted to synchronized changes in hormone levels or, to use the subway analogy, there are established frequencies of communication and well-worked-out rules of travel. In menopause, hormone levels become unpredictable, and the messages that once moved smoothly from the outer-borough vasomotor systems into the control-center hypothalamus become chaotic and imprecise.

Lessening estrogen sets the stage for hot flashes. It may also make the skin more sensitive to calibrations of heat, but estrogen is not the only trigger. Studies have found little variation between estrogen levels in women who do and do not flash. Dr. Naomi Rance, a professor of neurology at the University of Arizona, studied cells in the hypothalamus. She found that kisspeptin, neurokinin B, and dynorphin (KNDy) neurons were twice the size in menopausal women as they were in premenopausal ones. "They were large and overexcited," she told me. Using animal models, Dr. Rance found that these discharging neurons may be what brings on a flash. As heat is off-loaded, the heart rate increases, by seven to fifteen more beats per minute. Vasodilation permits warm blood to circulate quickly into the arms, thighs, and calves.

One study showed that the first part of the outer body to heat up was the fingertips.

A flash is both something going wrong and something going right. Hot flashes may ward off hardening of the arteries and plaque buildup associated with heart disease. And as the brain struggles to find equilibrium, it also grows more flexible. With each flash, the brain adjusts to a wider range of hormonal messages. Dr. Maki told me that recent studies have also shown that while it's trying to reset, the brain learns to make its own estrogen. Could the post-reproductive flexible brain be, in part, responsible for the resilience, wisdom, and peace I see in the older women I admire? "We don't know for sure," Maki said, "but it's definitely possible."

My bus moves, buoyant as a boat, past the Jersey strip malls, the neon liquor-store signs, the traffic-worn trees, 7-Elevens, Outback Steakhouses. A red lantern floats out of a Chinese restaurant's front window and hovers in the air over the wet street. Rain hits the big window and falls in blue streaks down the glass. We climb up into the mountains. Pass Bear Mountain. On Route 17, the lights get farther apart until it's just mottled darkness, the rain-smeared window, and the old man snoring gently beside me.

From my bag I pull out my Flash Count Diary. Eight flashes today so far. On the subway going under the East River the heat came on so fast I pulled off my coat and sweater and sat in my undershirt. I flashed while eating a Greek salad at a diner and while perusing a book on killer whales at Book Culture. I flashed at the Citibank where I got cash and in line at the coffee shop. The worst flash occurred while I was teaching. I felt the dart of panic as my face started to bake, and heat escaped through the top of my head. I kept talking, pretending nothing was wrong. When I shifted back in my chair, I saw the two dark wet spots on the table where my arms had been.

Near Monticello, in the foothills of the Catskills, the bus pulls off the highway and I see, through the rain, a gas station, blunt under the fluorescent light. A pale blonde woman pumps gas into her Jeep; a man inside gestures angrily at the cashier. The old man beside me wakes, pulls out his cell phone, punches in a number, and starts to talk. He's not sure. Is he going to die? The doctor was so vague. The old man is facing death. I am at the meridian, life's disconcerting center. Unease flows into my brain. I feel the first torrid prick and my heart thumps. I panic, desperate to break free of both my body and the reality of my own mortality. I pull off my sweater and press the inside of my wrist up against the bus window. The cool glass against my skin helps a little as I'm overtaken again by the ascending heat.

2 ● Free Lolita

When I read that female killer whales also go through menopause, I was coming off yet another sleepless night. I'd taken a break from the novel I was working on, a book about a woman who becomes unrecognizable to herself, to read the science section of *The New York Times*. Inside was a story, based on a scientific paper by Darren Croft and Emma Foster, on how, like human women, Southern Resident killer whales go through menopause and then have a long post-reproductive life. The older females not only live thirty to fifty years after menopause but they also lead their pods—complex cohesive family groups—particularly in times when salmon, their main food source, is scarce. Elder females have a plethora of ecological information and all whales, even younger males, choose to follow the post-reproductive females.

I went from the *Times* directly to YouTube and watched clip after clip of killer whales. Killer whales, or *Orcinus orca*, are the largest members of the dolphin family. They are as long as twenty-five feet and weigh up to seven tons. Their dorsal fins can reach six feet. Killer whales' brains are four times as big as our own and, like ours, have spindle cells that have been linked to empathy. Mothers raise one child at a time. They nurse for several years and teach their offspring to speak, forage, and follow the rituals of their pod.

I watched SeaWorld footage of Corky, a fifty-two-year-old post-reproductive female, on her back, waving her dorsal fins at the crowd. Katina, forty-one, slides herself onto a concrete ledge as part of a marine show. Lolita, fifty, swims tight laps around her small tank at the Miami Seaquarium. Wild whales live into old age, but in aquariums most die within five years. Lolita is the second-oldest whale in captivity and the only survivor of the Puget Sound capture of 1970, when Southern Resident whales were herded by boat, airplane, and explosives into nets. Lolita is an anomaly, moving into her forty-fifth year as a captive performer. Footage shows her swimming in her pool, the smallest orca tank in North America; its width is less than four lengths of her body, its depth less than one length. She swims frenetically from wall to wall, like an agitated soul trapped inside a concrete body.

◉ ◉ ◉

My favorite footage shows wild whales underwater. They are harder to see as they call to one another with clicks, squeaks, buzzes, donkey brays, and an unnerving sound like a human voice on helium. I watch them dive down so deep I can barely see them on my screen—it's as if they've moved down through my computer, through the top of my desk, and are hovering in the dark space below, just white patches in black water.

I listened continually for the Southern Residents near the San Juan Islands via the Lime Kiln hydrophone, an underwater microphone that streams live sound and records whale vocalizations as the orcas pass through Haro Strait. Mostly I hear boat motors, tide fetch, ebb, and flow. As I worked at my desk in Brooklyn, there was an overlay of sound from the Salish Sea, the whales' home waters. When I was sad, I'd double down, listening while also watching footage of the Southern Residents on YouTube or flipping through pictures of whale encounters at the Center for Whale Research website. The center, on San Juan Island in Washington State, has been studying the Southern Residents since 1978.

I began to dream of whales. In the first, a small calf beaches. I know she's young because her white patches are still orange. As I move closer to the body, the calf's black fluke rises in what appears to be a wave. For a while the whales that move through my sleeping head are intact but appear in incongruous places. A tall dorsal fin in the Delaware River, rising beside my inner tube. A pod breaching and spy-hopping in the upstate lake where I swim. In one dream, the whales are tiny—I'm startled to find one in my bowl of soup. Other times the killer whales are colossal, as big as a city bus but liquid, flowing, like oil over the roof of my house in Brooklyn.

One night the whales lose their definition, their specific physical characteristics, and are more like shining orbs hovering over the hardwood floor. They look like I feel when I am floating in a dream. The dream might have a different story line completely—say, my reoccurring one of being sent back to college to live in a dorm room—but the whales are still there, spots of energy wading over the grassy campus quad. Sometimes their energy shuts off and they fall to the ground, a mass of fetid blubber. In a recent dream, two whales were laid out in an L shape on my bed. I was confronted with the reality of their bodies, an intimacy so excruciating it was almost obscene.

The whales accompany me, not unlike other invisible presences: a boyfriend whose physical tenderness was hard to get out from under and, more recently, my mother, a phantom whose proximity both tears and quickens. The whales' presence is similar in sensation to—psychic pressure, sudden jerks at the edge of my eye—but different from being haunted by a person. The whales remain near but separate, unknown.

◉ ◉ ◉

When Lolita arrived at the Miami Seaquarium in 1970, another older whale was already living there. Hugo, a Southern Resident captured a few years earlier, was a large male with a collapsed dorsal fin. All male whales in captivity have collapsed dorsal fins, a sign of ill health from a diet of frozen fish and overly warm tank water. Hugo also suffered from zoochosis, self-destructively swimming over and over into the side of his concrete pool. Whale advocates believe he was suicidal. On her arrival, Lolita was named after Nabokov's unlucky heroine and "married" to the much older Hugo, a.k.a. Humbert. The two mated—once in the middle of a whale show—though Lolita never got pregnant.

I watched archival footage of skits that Lolita and Hugo performed over the years. In an early 1970s routine, Hugo goes up against the "boxer" Scrap Iron MacAtee. Scrap Iron comes out in a white robe, red silk shorts, and boxing gloves. Hugo, to taunt him, spins around with his tongue out. Scrap Iron gets into a small rowboat, which Hugo knocks over, and then he drags Scrap Iron to the side of the pool, where he is down for the count. As the announcer counts backward from ten, Lolita, who has been hiding, rises up and splashes water on Scrap Iron. The two whales do a victory lap around the pool, then jump up together, reaching their noses twenty feet in the air to touch two balls suspended over the water.

In 1980 Hugo was successful in killing himself. He died after swimming violently into the concrete wall of his tank. The attending veterinarian, Dr. Jesse R. White, wrote in his necropsy report that Hugo died of an aneurysm of a cerebellar artery.

After Hugo's death, Lolita continued on alone. In one film from the 1980s, her trainer rides her in nearly every position imaginable. Standing on her back, holding on to her dorsal fin as if Lolita were a surfboard, lying on her back, lying on her white belly in a human-animal embrace. The trainer stands on Lolita's snout, as she shoots him up and out of the water. The trainer sits on Lolita's head and he is again shot up out of the water. In one routine, as the trainer stands on Lolita's back and she swims, her tail flapping with exaggerated movements like a giant bath toy, one, two, three dolphins jump onto her and ride her, along with the trainer, as if Lolita were a flatbed boat.

◎ ◎ ◎

I became obsessed with Lolita. I read blogs about her and joined Facebook pages committed to her release. I searched Miami library websites for early Seaquarium footage. She was a kindred menopausal creature I felt unreasonably drawn to. "I desperately wanted to be close to animals," writes Charles Foster in his 2016 book, *Being a Beast*. "Part of this was the conviction that they knew something that I didn't and that I, for unexamined reasons, needed to know."

So with no real plan I flew down to Miami from New York. I wanted to be near a postmenopausal whale, and to protest, along with animal rights activists, for her freedom.

◎ ◎ ◎

The Miami Seaquarium could be considered kitsch, with its 1960s space-age concrete architecture and chipped pastel paint, but it's too sinister, more Floridian Gothic. A scuba diver scrubs crud off the glass from inside the giant aquarium, a skull flag flies over the pirate-themed playground, and a sea turtle with what looks like algae growing over its back floats glumly in a bathtub-size tank.

In the killer whale stadium, with its carnival-sideshow vibe, Michael Jackson's "Black or White" blares over the speakers, and three trainers in wet suits walk out onto the concrete platform. The young women smile and wave. Lolita's tank seems even smaller in person, not much bigger than a backyard swimming pool. It's hard to believe a creature as big as a van, used to swimming a hundred miles a day, must remain in this barren concrete pit. This is the first show of the day, and from reading about whales that live in sea parks, I know that Lolita is hungry. They keep her hungry so she will do her tricks. A trainer with a long braid down her back makes a sharp hand signal, and Lolita swims to the front of the tank and twists up from the water. Spray flies off her gigantic, glittering body, and the crowd cheers.

————

The large screen behind the tank lights up, showing footage of L pod, Lolita's family, as they swim free in the Salish Sea. Lolita rests with her chin on the concrete as a recorded voice tells about the endangered Southern Residents. Lolita appears to be watching the screen; maybe she knows that when the movie is over, she will get another chunk of fish, but maybe she remembers her family. I had read that Hyak, the captive whale used in the marine scientist John Ford's 1980s echolocation study, knocked his head often against the observational glass to signal that he wanted researchers to show him the picture book made up of images of his wild relatives.

The calls Lolita continues to make have been identified as L pod vocalizations. One scientist speculates that she may not comprehend she's three thousand miles from her home waters. Lolita may think the Salish Sea is just over the Seaquarium's jumbotron.

"The question that truly occupies [animals]," writes J. M. Coetzee in *The Lives of Animals*, "as it occupies the rat and the cat and every other animal trapped in the hell of laboratory or zoo, is: Where is home and how do I get there?"

After the film is over, Lolita waves with her pectoral fins and slaps her tail. Each time the crowd claps, Lolita heads back to her trainer for a fish. Finally the trainer, looking bored, feeding Lolita with one hand and sipping on a Slurpee straw with the other, shoots her hand down and then straight up. Lolita plunges underwater. She is gone for several minutes before she launches up and completely out of the water, her body hovering over the blue. Her breach is akin to a biblical miracle, a spectacle my eyes see but that my brain can't absorb. The crowd is silent as she lands in an upward cascade of liquid lace.

Breach: (1) A broken, ruptured, or torn condition. (2) A gap (as in a wall) made by battering. (3) A leap, especially of a whale out of the water.

◉ ◉ ◉

To be stuck in a small cramped place, to wait for outside intervention. Is it stupid to compare my captivity to Lolita's? Is it insensitive to actual captives, real prisoners? Yes. But it does not negate that while I am not in a tank, cage, or cell, I have felt my menopausal world shrinking, my freedom decreasing. "For I have missed the feeling," the poet Laurie Sheck writes in her book *Captivity*, "of being able to go somewhere else, / Delicately barred as I am / In this slow conversion of myself into nothingness."

I have struggled with why Lolita's captivity feels familiar to me. Why I find her dilemma so compelling. I recognize the feeling of being held captive, not literally, like Lolita, but metaphorically. A female captivity always binding but that, without fertility, tightens further. I am restricted, stuck in the box the greater culture uses to enclose and reduce older women. Lolita must be what the Seaquarium defines, a creature who does not want to be free, a prisoner who must be grateful to her captors, a female who does tricks in order to be fed.

◎ ◎ ◎

As the crowd cheers and Lolita swims back to her trainer, I wonder if she's feeling sorry for us, her spectators. It's clear there is something wrong with us. We are, on some level, blind. I wonder, as I watch Lolita rest her chin on the concrete, if she is enraged, as all captives are at first. Or if she feels, as some women do after years of captivity, a misplaced gratitude.

Captivity from the Latin *captivitas*, means "bondage," often in the sense of a person held by the enemy during war. It also means "blindness." Captives are commonly blindfolded, but the captor also experiences a sort of moral blindness. I wanted to get close to another menopausal creature, but I see that Lolita's captivity, while bringing her closer physically, actually makes it impossible for me to get an authentic sense of her, to *see* her at all.

After the show, techno music hammers, and Lolita logs by the side of the tank. She floats with her eyes closed against the sharp chlorine. It's terrible to see her lying lifeless, but better than an earlier bit when she was trained to "catch" the kisses spectators threw at her. Ken Balcomb, the founder of the Center for Whale Research, thinks Lolita suffers from Stockholm syndrome. She is bonded to people who deny her freedom. In this way she's not unlike heroines in human-captivity narratives; in order to survive in an unspeakable environment, she must establish a long-term relationship with her captor. Some advocates assume that Lolita's compliance is chemical—that she's on both tranquilizers and antidepressants. Her suffering as a creature torn from the wild and alone in her small watery cell is palpable. People push in, hold their cell phones above their heads, and smile.

◎ ◎ ◎

The next day, I stand in front of the Seaquarium with twenty other protesters and try to turn away cars. From where we rally, alongside the Rickenbacker Causeway, we can see across the parking lot to the Seaquarium entrance as well as the concrete backside of the killer whale stadium. The sun is roasting. I can already feel my shoulders burning and the skin of my face getting stiff. With a bullhorn, a protester shouts, "Educate yourself!" in both English and Spanish. Others pass out xeroxed literature about Lolita's captivity and the plan to release her back into her home waters in Washington State. A young man in a VEGAN T-shirt holds up a hand-lettered sign: LEAVE ANIMALS THE FUCK

ALONE. Two young women are in orca costumes, black hoods lined with pink, their generous sleeves as pectoral fins. A little boy named Juan protests with his family. He has drawn a picture of Lolita and written above it: EXTRAÑO A MI MAMA!

Not all protesters want the same thing. Some want Lolita to be retired to a sea pen in her home waters in Washington State. Others just want her to be allowed to rest, to not have to perform in show after show every day of the week. One woman wants the Seaquarium to build an overhang so Lolita can have some relief from the blazing Floridian sun that cracks and dries her skin. A few protesters don't believe Lolita will be released but hope, by letting people know about her suffering, to turn public opinion against cetacean captivity. Not all the protesters are young. An older Russian man holds a picture of Saint Francis with lettering that reads SHE HAS A SOUL TOO. His name is Oleg. "Once you can feel for the animals," he tells me, "you are really in the world of the air and the water and the butterflies, not just down here trying to make a living."

◎ ◎ ◎

I want Lolita's story to end in escape and deliverance. I want her released back to her home waters in Washington State. She went on a long journey, underwent extraordinary ordeals and humiliations. Now she must return home and be reunited with her family. Without reconciliation, there is no closure. Even if she is released, there is no telling if she'll be able to overcome her captivity. After eighteen years of being held captive in a backyard shed, Jaycee Dugard continues to be haunted by her loneliness. "Today I sometimes struggle," she writes in her book *A Stolen Life*, "with feelings of loneliness even when I am not alone . . . Hours turned into days, days to weeks, and weeks to months and then years."

At the very least, activists hope to force the Seaquarium to build Lolita a bigger tank, a legal-size one. In recent years the U.S. Department of Agriculture has finally acknowledged what supporters have known: Lolita's tank does not meet all space requirements set by the 1966 Animal Welfare Act. It is too small. PETA filed a motion to strip Seaquarium of its license to display large mammals. Seaquarium responded as it does each time activists press for Lolita's release. In a statement, Andrew Hertz, the Seaquarium director, emphasizes her age: "The approximately 50-year-old post-reproductive Lolita . . ." He goes on to list the ocean's many dangers, implying that the sea is too wild a place for the over-the-hill female whale. Hertz seems unaware that post-reproductive matriarchs pilot their pods. They are neither frail nor apprehensive but in every way leaders of their communities. Whales much older than Lolita command their pods in the Salish Sea. Ocean Sun, an eighty-five-year-old whale believed to be Lolita's mother, is one of the leaders of L pod. And a whale fifty years Lolita's senior, the 104-year-old matriarch known as J2, or Granny, guides the J, K, and L pods.

◎ ◎ ◎

What was happening to me was hard to explain to other people. Whenever I tried, I found that language failed, that I could not explain how the whales had both infiltrated me and given me hope. I felt bewildered. I'd always been suspicious of animal-obsessed people, like the PETA girl on the subway who once shoved the corpse of an electrocuted fox in my face. How do you explain you've been enchanted by a creature, an apex predator? I felt like the Maori girl in the film *Whale Rider*. The film alternates between footage of whales swimming underwater and the girl, Paikea, struggling on land with Koro, her grandfather. Koro does not believe girls can lead. The relationship between girl and whale is subtle, delicate. Paikea must ultimately ride a whale in order to convince her family, her community, and herself that she possesses both essential wildness and strength.

It was all so embarrassing. I am not Native American. I am not even a girl. Though I am a female in the midst of a crossing. I am a fifty-three-year-old woman, an urban person on the back side of middle age, drawn for the first time in my life to an animal, to Lolita, but also to J2, the Southern Resident matriarch, Granny. I watch footage of J2 playing with a dolphin, of her breaching and spy-hopping with her family after a salmon feed, of her swimming beside younger pod members, staying close to them, as if giving advice.

❀ ❀ ❀

"Storylessness," writes the feminist Katha Pollitt in her foreword to Carolyn Heilbrun's book *Writing a Woman's Life*, "has been women's biggest problem." Heilbrun felt that women have been confined to erotic narratives and that a common cultural understanding leads to the altar. Our story ends with a house, babies, a loving husband. "This story," Pollitt writes, "not only fails to fill a lifetime, it puts the plot line in the hands of others, men who do or do not admire, love, offer marriage and make full female adulthood possible."

Menopause, with its loss of fertility, its dislocation, frays the narrative further. I have felt that my story was over, that nothing more would happen to me. Unless, of course, I divorced again and the old marriage plot could be invigorated, albeit with less sex appeal and lower stakes. But what if the postmenopausal narrative, like the prepubescent one, is focused not on romance, but on a creature? Like the stories I loved at twelve, *Charlotte's Web*, *Misty of Chincoteague*, and *The Lion, the Witch and the Wardrobe*. I am not interested in girl meets boy, but in woman meets whale. "Questing," Pollitt writes, "is what makes a woman the hero of her own life."

3 ● The Animals

Long before Darwin uncovered the evolutionary forces that linked us to animals, menopause itself was associated with the ineffable, the bestial, the base. A French medieval alchemist explained that if you took a hair from an old woman's mons pubis, mixed it with menses, and planted it in a dung heap, "at the end of the year you'd find a wicked venomous beast." Edward Tilt, the author of the popular 1857 book *The Change of Life in Health and Disease*, associated the change with violent behaviors, drinking binges, stealing, suicide attempts, and recklessness with money. One of his patients, he claimed, believed the devil had lodged inside her womb. "Something is sent to the brain," he wrote, "so that women are no longer the mistresses of their own actions, she is fuddled with animal spirits." Tilt, a medical educator and member of the Royal College of Physicians, wrote that hot flashes were preceded by "strange sensations, which resemble pulses, like a live animal throbbing in the stomach."

One of my menopausal correspondents wrote to me: "Reporting that I finally get the whole animal thing regarding menopause, suddenly my physical body is very present. Heart palpitations. Strange bloating. Shape shifting like a motherfucker."

The anthropologist Ernest Becker has written that menopause is an "animal birthday," a reminder of our "creatureliness." Other animal birthdays for woman are menstruation and birth, but both, unlike menopause, come with captivating and all-consuming new worlds. Sexual desire rises with menstruation, along with physical pleasure, intimacy, the vagaries of romantic relationships. Birth brings the transformation of motherhood; our brains are reworked so that a new and tiny person's needs supplant our own.

Only menopause arrives without absorbing directives. Instead of new obsessions and responsibilities I feel a nothingness, a negation. It's a void created in part by an oversexed patriarchal culture that has little room for older women. The message, never stated directly but manifesting in myriad ways, is an overwhelmingly nihilistic one: Your usefulness is over. Please step to the sidelines. Counterpart to inner emptiness is an outer invisibility. One woman told me that after she turned fifty, she felt herself becoming more invisible each day. In the novel *Calling Invisible Woman,* Jeanne Ray writes about Clover, a fifty-four-year-old housewife who discovers that a pharmaceutical combination of hormone replacements, calcium tablets, antidepressants, and Botox has made her and other women her age literally invisible. The novel's real horror is not the invisibility itself, but that no one, not even her husband, notices that she is missing.

In turning to animals, I wanted to study a few female mammals in middle age, hoping they might be a conduit to what the philosopher William James, in one of his lectures, called the "more." I'm not sure if menopause, with all its needling, exhausting symptoms, triggered or exacerbated the dark feelings of spiritual malaise I started to have at fifty. But I found the texture of my soul not Melville's damp and drizzly November but a cold and newsprint-y March. I less wanted to knock off people's hats than I, in my loneliness, wanted to touch strangers' hair.

Becoming animal. This does not mean I go feral or become base. It is not complicated. If you pay attention, you can feel animal many times a day: when you fuck, shit, breastfeed your baby, run, swim, eat, or have a hot flash. But I find it hard to sit in the void with my animal self. I want to check my phone every few minutes, to make sure I have enough soy milk for my morning coffee, to see how many people liked the picture I posted on Facebook of my cat.

Menstruation brings thoughts of the beastly to the writer Carmen Maria Machado. "I think of my body as an animal," she writes, "one that perpetually needs more than I can give her." Menopause, too, brings the sense of being animal. As one woman breaks into a full-body sweat at a parent-teacher conference, she feels like "a trapped animal." Another feels like she's finally able to accept her corporeal form: "I am conscious that I am and have always been an animal." There is the woman who thinks of her hot flashes as honey badgers, as in the social media meme "honey badger don't care." Many women associate a new don't-give-a-fuck quality with the animal. For most, including myself, a sense of the animal is connected to mortality—that we are creatures inside a life cycle. For the first time, I feel I have a time stamp, an expiration date.

◉ ◉ ◉

Nothing quite prepares you for the sight of an elephant up close. Ambika, the sixty-eight-year-old, post-reproductive female I've come to visit at the National Zoo, is like a swatch of a dream ripped out and pasted into my flat and ordinary reality. When she opens her mouth, her breath makes a big cloud of condensation in the cold air. She reaches her trunk up, the tip wet and pink like a toothless second mouth, and sniffs my shoes, my shoulder, my hair.

———

For weeks, in anticipation of this visit, I've been watching YouTube videos of Ambika delighting crowds with sprays of water and by throwing dirt up onto her back. I've read her biography, researched by her keeper Maria Galloway: how she was captured in 1959, at age eleven, in the Coorg forest in India, trained by a mahout in an elephant camp, and shipped to the United States on a steamer. When she caught a cold during the crossing, she was given, along with her usual hay, a fifth of bourbon and a ten-pound bag of onions.

Galloway points out signs of age: Ambika's bony protruding forehead, her frayed cabbage-leaf ears, how she drags her right foot because of arthritis in the ankle. She's smaller than the other elephants, delicate, even frail. Her energy is centered, though, steady and intense, unlike that of the young bull who, with his trunk, continuously rattles the gate lock.

It's this gravity that in the wild gives older female elephants their edge. Matriarchs lead their family groups to food and water and dig wells in times of drought. They are skillful listeners. Phyllis Lee, an elephant researcher at the University of Stirling, found that the older the matriarch, the longer she listened to audio recordings and the better she was at deciphering the unique sounds of other elephant groups, as well as distinguishing the roar of female lions from that of the more dangerous male lions. Karen Mccomb, another elephant researcher, found that matriarchs also distinguish between tribes. When played a recording of phrases of the elephant-hunting Maasai tribe, the matriarch signaled for her family to form a defensive bunch, while phrases from the Kuba, a tribe that does not hunt elephants, elicited no response at all.

Across animal species, both menopause and post-reproductive life are not common. Some female insects and fish have short but heroic post-reproductive lives. Salmon, as is well known, die after swimming upriver to spawn. Research has shown that those females who live for even an extra day can protect their eggs from predators. The adactylidium mite mother makes the ultimate sacrifice, as her young hatch inside her body and eat their way out. My favorite is the social aphid. After she is finished reproducing, this tiny she-warrior pulls off her wings and sets herself up to guard the mouth of her nest, where her daughters now breed. When an intruder tries to break in, like the flailing ladybug larva I watched on YouTube, the post-reproductive female throws herself at the predator and, using wax she secretes from her abdomen, latches her small self to the larva's mouth.

Studies concerning the later-life fertility of elephants and gorillas are ongoing. Their fecundity diminishes with age, but unlike that of killer whales and human women, their fertility does not cease completely and is not followed by many years of post-reproductive life. Menopause remains one of the great mysteries of biology. It goes against the theory of natural selection—that a creature's main focus must be having as many offspring as possible. Menopause is an enigma, a physical characteristic that should, according to Darwin's theory, have been selected against.

At the zoo, Galloway tells me, they take no chances on their inhabitants' fertility. All the other female elephants, except for Ambika, are on birth control. At sixty-eight she could technically still be cycling. In the wild, elephants as old as sixty have been known to give birth, after a gestation period that lasts twenty-two months, and most live six to twelve years after their last baby was born. Their post-reproductive life is short but rich. They not only lead the greater herd but also help their individual offspring. A recent study found that the older the matriarch, the longer her daughters lived and the higher their reproductive rates.

Ambika's reproductive history is straightforward. She has never had a calf. When she turned fifty, blood clots were found in her uterus—a condition similar to endometriosis in women. Her keepers decided to use hormone blockers to shut down her reproductive organs. My questions about Ambika's sex life are answered frankly. Maybe it's the trauma of captivity, Galloway says, but Ambika has never been mounted by a bull. Never even shown signs, as some of the other females have, of masturbating.

Ambika, like any creature who has lived into her sixties, has a long emotional history to go along with her biological one. While there is no way to know exactly how Ambika feels, Galloway has written about what she has witnessed. Elephants bond for companionship and emotional support. These friendships can last a lifetime. When her current bond mate Shanthi's calf died, Ambika remained constantly by the grieving mother's side. When Toni, another elephant friend, died, she spent time with the body, caressing Toni's head with her trunk. Most heart-wrenching was Ambika's fit of grief over the dead body of her first bond mate, Shanti (without an *h*), as she was cut up with a chain saw and removed piece by piece from an adjoining stall. "Ambika became very distressed," Galloway writes in a zookeepers' newsletter. "She acted out to the point keepers thought she was not safe and needed to be moved. They had to walk her past Shanti's body to get her to another place further away. For many years after, Ambika refused to walk into a stall unless another elephant walked in front of her."

◎ ◎ ◎

"A lot of people ask," the primate researcher Sue Margulis tells me, "if the post-reproductive gorillas are grumpy." While she and her team can check hormone levels, there is no way for them to assess if the older gorillas are physically uncomfortable, no way to tell if they endure menopausal symptoms like moodiness or hot flashes. "At one point we thought of aiming a laser gun at them to see if their temperature was fluctuating." The technology for this experiment was never perfected.

Margulis, who teaches at Canisius College in Buffalo, New York, and spends mornings studying gorillas, tells me there is still considerable controversy surrounding the question of menopause in nonhuman primates. She and her research partner, over the past twenty years, tested the hormone levels in thirty older female gorillas living in zoos across North America.

Several times a month, keepers collected fecal matter, packed it in dry ice, and mailed it to Margulis, who tested the waste for hormone levels. Most of the females were living in potential breeding situations with their silverback, a sexually mature male with a thick coat of silver-gray back hair. In the wild, gorillas live in harems with one silverback male to several females. Their menstrual cycle is much like humans', lasting about thirty days. Estrus, or the time during which females can become pregnant, lasts two to three days. During that fertile time, keepers also took note of when the females masturbated, inspected their genitals, or gave their silverback what is known as "the look," the one that says in no uncertain terms, *I want sex*.

What Margulis found was that "menopause" in gorillas, while slightly more pronounced than in elephants, is not as clear-cut as menopause in humans. Hormone levels do drop, and, like women, gorillas also become less fertile with age. Margulis tells me that part of the reason it's so hard to be certain about primate menopause is that in the wild, most females die before they stop cycling. Quality of life for the older females is grim. Female dominance depends on having babies, so once a female stops reproducing, she falls to the lowest rung of the social ladder. "They lose interest in the silverback," Margulis says, "and the silverback loses interest in them." Just like humans, gorillas suffer from arthritis and osteoporosis, but the thing that often kills them is starvation. Once their teeth rot and they can no longer chew, they starve.

Dian Fossey writes in her book *Gorillas in the Mist* about a few older females she studied in the forests of Rwanda. Near the end of shy Idanno's life, her silverback, Beethoven, slows his group's pace to keep up with her, and in the last days of her life, though his group has younger females, he carefully builds his night nest of leaves and branches and invites the elderly female to sleep beside him. Even more compelling is the partnership of silverback Rafiki and Coco. Coco is Rafiki's only female. Coco, Fossey writes, has deep wrinkles on her face, a balding head and rump, a graying muzzle, and flabby, hairless upper arms. She is missing many teeth. One day, while Fossey watches, Rafiki notices that Coco has fallen behind.

He stops his group and waits. When Coco approaches, they gaze deeply into each other's eyes before throwing their arms around each other's backs and walking together up the slope. The two also share a night nest and "resemble a gracefully aging old married couple."

While Ambika is the oldest living elephant in captivity, and Lolita is the second-oldest orca, Colo, at age fifty-nine, is the oldest captive gorilla. Audra Meinelt, the assistant primate curator of the Columbus Zoo, believes that Colo is no longer cycling. She does not give "the look" to her silverback or to her male keepers. Neither Meinelt nor her coworkers have ever seen a gorilla menstruate. There is no labia swelling, like there is with other primates, and blood is absorbed and hidden by the animals' thick, dark fur.

Colo, as the first gorilla born in captivity, had a long and celebrated life at the zoo before, at age forty-five, she started to distance herself from her family. In the mornings when the family left their private sleeping quarters, Colo held back, signaling to her keepers she wanted to be alone. Colo's new enclosure is next to her family's, and she still makes clear, by vocalizing and running back and forth, when she disapproves of something the silverback does. Meinelt feels that Colo may have gotten tired of her silverback's "theatrics."

These days Colo moves a little slower. The steps to her habitat have been changed to ramps, and along with her regular diet, she is given cranberry juice for urinary tract infections and whole grains to battle constipation. On her fifty-ninth birthday, while spectators sing to her, Colo runs a finger through her birthday cake's frosting, brings it to her nose, and sniffs. Under her deep-set brown eyes, the skin is wrinkled, and the hair on her head is silvered. Her fans want her to open her presents, but it's clear, as Colo pulls down the color-ful paper chains and drapes them around her neck, that she isn't going to rush for anyone.

◎ ◎ ◎

Even though menopause has pushed me back onto my ani-mal frame, I don't kid myself that now I am one with them. In the presence of animals, I am thrilled by their physicality. But I also feel their deep inscrutability. "Nothing, as a matter of fact," Georges Bataille writes, "is more closed to us than this animal life from which we are descended." He felt the only way to speak of it overtly was through a poetry that slips toward the unknown. The writer Lydia Millet also warns against shallow interspecies enlightenment and claims that the fact we cannot fathom animals is a great and precious gift: "I cherish the reality that other animals are us, in that they have sentience and are not us, in that the nature of that sentience is an eternal mystery."

In *Break of Day*, Colette's 1928 novel, the main character, also named Colette, agrees that no matter how much time goes by, animals remain mysterious. "The passage of the centuries never bridges the chasm which yawns between them and man." As she ages, though, and moves into menopause, her sympathy with animals increases. "When I enter a room where you're alone with your animals," her former husband tells her, "I feel I'm being indiscreet. One of these days you'll retire to a jungle." She is attuned to animal emotion: "The tragedies of birds in the air, the subterranean combats of rodents, the suddenly increased sound of a swan on the warpath, the hopeless look of horses and donkeys are so many messages addressed to me." Colette claims, at the age of fifty-four, that she no longer wants to marry a man. "But I still dream that I am marrying a very big cat."

● ● ●

On my fifty-fourth birthday I get up early and drive through the Bronx, past Westchester, to Lucky Orphans Horse Rescue in Dover Plains, New York. Winter is sliding into spring; the trees are in first bud. Once I turn onto Route 22, tulips bob in yards, and tiny white petals, like confetti, float down over the road.

I've come to meet yet another post-reproductive creature, less exotic than elephants or gorillas. A horse. A thoroughbred, no less, with the official name of Overdue Number. Her sanctuary name is Willow. To my eye, she's the prettiest horse in her all-female herd—a half dozen mares in a field standing around a small barn with a tin roof. Many of her herdmates have far more horrific stories than Willow's. Cadbury was rescued from a summer camp. Her owners never took off her bridle, so it grew into her snout. The foal Tulla has scars all over her body from a mountain lion attack.

Willow isn't the oldest horse at the sanctuary, but her biological predicament is closest to my own. She is here because she is no longer a viable breeder. Born in 2002 in Virginia, Willow raced only once before being sold in 2007 as a broodmare. Broodmares are bred each year and, like Premarin mares, whose urine is used to make hormone supplements, are kept continuously pregnant. Willow's offspring included Penalty Due, Celestial Number, Vision and Prayer, Noon Shadow 3, and Thunder Thief.

In February 2016, Willow miscarried, and her owners decided her body was no longer viable for reproduction. When horse owners decide their horses are no longer useful, either for riding, racing, or breeding, they send them to auction. But it's a fantasy that older horses are cared for after their usefulness has passed. Most are not bought at auction and are sold to the slaughterhouse.

Death is the hardest part of feeling animal. "In every calm and reasonable person," Philip Roth writes, "there is a hidden second person scared witless about death." As a human, I view myself as a significant being who will persist, at least symbolically, after I am gone, but to be animal is to die a forgettable death. Animals look particularly dead splayed along the highway, lumps of fur in puddles of inky blood. Menopause has aggravated my sense of entrapment and death, uncovering what, for so long, I have struggled to deny.

Deanna Mancuso, the founder of the sanctuary, says that Willow was depressed when she first arrived. Her ears, alert in healthy horses, had flipped over. She wasn't eating and had no interest in people or other horses. An article in *Reiner* magazine, the publication of the National Reining Horse Association, lays out the criteria for reproduction at broodmare farms. A mare is culled if one of her foals is not easily trainable, if she has trouble in labor, if the money from the sale of her foals does not equal her upkeep, or if, like Willow, she becomes subfertile and requires too much medical care. The article sneers at "welfare programs" that crop up when owners become emotionally connected to their older mares.

Before I leave Lucky Orphans, Willow lowers her head and presses her warm check to my face. Her eyelashes brush my forehead, and I see, like a tiny rain cloud, the milky cataract floating in her eye. Mancuso tells me how, surrounded by mares her own age, Willow seems to be getting over her miscarriage and adjusting to life at the sanctuary. She's become a surrogate mother to Tulla, the foal attacked by a mountain lion. She lets her dry nurse and shows her disapproval, by whinnying and stomping, when the foal misbehaves.

◎ ◎ ◎

Lolita. Ambika. Colo. Willow. Their animal spirits reside in their animal bodies and my animal spirit resides in mine. I have tried to understand what their post-reproductive life is actually like. I have mostly failed. I read book after book about animals, studying their habits and wishing I could be wilder. But I also struggle to accept that I too am a biological creature no different from a whale or a horse. I long to comprehend animals just as much as my ancestors did, the first humans who crawled into the earth and painted animal-human creatures on cave walls. "There is every indication that the first men were closer than we are to the animal world," writes Georges Bataille. "They distinguished the animals from themselves perhaps, but not without a feeling of doubt mixed with terror and longing."

4 ● Mind at the End of Its Tether

In Paris, where I teach each July, they don't believe in air-conditioning. I flash every hour, like a junkie, jonesing not for heroin but for hormones. Besides flashes, I am dealing with insomnia and anxiety. When I wake in the night, my fingers tremble as I reach for the water glass on the side table. In the early mornings the temperature is in the high seventies. If I stay in the shade at the Luxembourg Gardens near the circle of stone queens, the heat does not yet blot out coherent thought. But as the temperature climbs into the eighties and then the nineties, Paris, with its cream-colored buildings, floral effusions, and rows of café tables lined with wicker-back chairs, becomes a furnace.

Evenings, after a day of teaching in a sweltering classroom, I sit on the couch in the fifth-floor garret apartment, trying to write comments on student papers. I feel the emotional blitz, as if I've been caught in a lie, and then comes fear. "I experienced a strong feeling of fear," William Burroughs writes in his book *Junky*. "I had the feeling that some horrible image was beyond the field of vision, moving, as I turned my head, so that I never quite saw it."

Back in Brooklyn, even in the air-conditioning and with the cool gel pillow pressed against my stomach, my body craves estrogen. But my brain does not get the estrogen it longs for and so, in sorrow and revolt, sends heat speeding along my nerves. I imagine the Pentecostal flame wavering just above my head.

The spirit, unlike the Father and Son of the Trinity, is more female, appearing only after the body is broken, permeable. The theologian Rudolf Bultmann has written that the Holy Spirit has two main manifestations: the animistic and the dynamistic. In the animistic, "an independent agent . . . can fall upon a man and take possession of him, enabling him or compelling him to perform manifestations of power." In the dynamistic, the spirit "appears as an impersonal force which fills a man like a fluid." When my husband, wanting a break from what he calls the arctic air-conditioning, cracks the window to let in the summer warmth, I feel a stream of sultry moist air move in, curl around the room, and hover over the bed.

———

I can't sleep. I have trouble both getting to sleep and staying asleep. As with so much in menopause, scientists don't know why some women have trouble sleeping. It may have something to do with lessening estrogen, but no study is conclusive. I lie in the dark feeling as De Quincey did when he was in opium withdrawal, as if a hundred years had gone by in a single night. I lie on my side but then throw off the sheet and lie on my back, pull up my nightgown, and hold the gel pillow against my bare chest. I watch out my bedroom window; hot wind rushes through the leaves, turning them to their silver sides. Summer is claustrophobic, the months in which, as De Quincy claimed, "the exuberant and riotous prodigity of life naturally forces the mind more powerfully up onto the antagonistic thoughts of death."

There is a difference, of course, between my withdrawal and a junkie's. The substance my body craves is not outside myself, not snorted or injected with a needle, but made by my own organs. My hormones diminish naturally, completely beyond my control. Some scientists say menopause is triggered when the number of viable eggs in the ovaries is too low; others admit they don't know why egg maturation stops and hormones diminish. Without hormones, my body changes again, just as it did in adolescence when I was flooded with estrogen and began to menstruate. While menstruation still carries stigma in our culture—we are *on the rag* and considered unstable because of fluctuating hormones—the fertile years of a woman's life are also considered her most essential. Menopause, on the other hand, is disparaged, even considered shameful. No one proposes we eliminate childhood, adolescence, or adulthood from the female life cycle. Only menopause is considered something to be cured and reversed, done away with completely.

Another way my dilemma is different from a junkie's is that a junkie's withdrawal, while uncomfortable, even excruciating, is considered necessary, a period of fire that leads to a more harmonious and balanced life. But many scientists, doctors, authors, and celebrities see the hormonal change as unnecessary, even old-fashioned. They would medicate my withdrawal, pushing me back on to hormones, back into menstruating, back into the docile, wet-pussied woman of an earlier phase.

In her book *The Sexy Years*, Suzanne Somers interviews Rita, a seventy-year-old woman who is on bioidentical hormones and still menstruates. Rita tells Somers all the things she wants to hear: "I have a youthful energy." She and her husband are "having a ball!" Before she went on hormones, Rita was starting to feel like she was living in someone else's body, alienated from herself. Then Dr. Schwarzbein, Somers's hormone doctor, told Rita about hormone therapy. "He explained to me that having a period is the most natural way to go through this passage."

Literature is rich with stories of men remaking women. There's *Pygmalion*, of course, and its progeny *My Fair Lady*. In

Hawthorne's *The Birthmark*, Aylmer loves science as much as he loves his wife, Georgiana. He longs to, using poison, remove the birthmark, the small red hand like a tiny splash of menstrual blood on his wife's cheek. After the operation Aylmer is ecstatic. "My peerless bride, it is successful! You are perfect!" But his wife understands what she's lost in her complicity with her husband's search for perfection: "You have rejected the best that the earth could offer." The story ends with the "perfect woman pass[ing] into the atmosphere" and an acknowledgment that the imperfection of the birthmark "was the bond by which an angelic spirit kept itself in union with a mortal frame."

Alymer has much in common with Dr. Robert Wilson, the author of *Feminine Forever*, the 1966 book that began American women's obsession with hormone supplements. The book sold 100,000 copies in its first seven months after publication. While examining a new fifty-five-year-old patient, a woman who's thin and pleasant, with soft skin, Wilson realizes that hormone replacement therapy could free women from menopause, keep them from witnessing "the death of their own womanhood."

To Wilson, menopause is a disease: "Menopause—far from being an act of fate or a state of mind—is in fact a deficiency disease." He believes a lack of estrogen not only ruins the female body—"breasts become flabby and shrink"—but also destroys the personality: "The transformation, within a few years, of a formerly pleasant, energetic woman into a dull-minded but sharp-tongued caricature of her former self is one of the saddest of human spectacles."

Most distressing to Wilson of menopausal symptoms is the dry, unyielding vagina. Dr. Frankenstein–like, Wilson tells us that "few processes in the entire body are as dramatic as the estrogenic transformation of the vagina." Under his careful care, one old woman found that her "pathologically dry, unyielding vagina had changed into a perfectly normal, supple, and resilient duct."

Wilson seems genuinely afraid of postmenopausal women, as if we were penis-repelling monsters: "The mere fact that such woman castrates are prevalent—and getting more so every day as the world fills up with older women—does not make it biologically natural."

Long before Wilson, doctors and scientists were bewildered by both menstruation and menopause. Aristotle thought a woman's cycle was caused by "nova luna repurget," the lunar cycle's pull on all liquid, be it ocean waters or uterine blood. Hippocrates speculated that women let unneeded blood go each month because they were less active than men. Pliny felt the odor of menstrual blood caused new wine to go sour and made seeds sterile, buds fall off trees, and iron corrode.

———

Early menopausal treatments were equally clueless. Never eat sausage, particularly before bed. Sponge the body three times a day with aromatic vinegar. Apply several leeches to the anus. Fast on milk one day out of every fifteen. Drink the bone marrow of recently killed animals. Get a transfusion of dog's blood. Even with treatment, these early books warn, menopausal women may become so sexually aroused they become prostitutes. They might also turn to the same sex for physical comfort. Some women will collect first one, then two, then a dozen cats. In the Q&A at the back of Edward Tilt's *The Change of Life in Health and Disease*, a woman asks if now that she's stopped menstruating, she'll bleed from other places on her body. Tilt answers that, yes, she may bleed monthly from her mouth or her nose.

The recommendations from *Woman's Change of Life*, published in 1958, one of the few early books on menopause written by a woman, gives more moderate advice. During the change, advises Dr. Isabel Hutton, husbands should give their wives their own bank accounts. Financial independence is soothing, as is moderate exercise and spa-like relaxation techniques. Women are instructed to lie on their beds and pretend to swim for twenty minutes before taking a soothing pine bath and then wrapping themselves in a warm, attractive dressing gown.

◉ ◉ ◉

Ovariin, introduced by Merck drugs in 1899, was the first official hormone supplement. Ovariin was a brown powder made from the dried and pulverized ovaries of cows. It was reputed to lessen the menopausal symptoms of hot flashes and night sweats. After mixing it with water, women drank down their daily supplement. Before and during Ovariin's rise in popularity, other cruder and more extreme hormonal treatments were used by both men and women. One aging doctor experimented with hormones on himself. In the 1920s, Dr. Charles-Édouard Brown-Séquard, a seventy-two-year-old neurologist and member of the Royal Society of London, made a rejuvenation liquid out of testicular blood, semen, and the juice extracted from the crushed testicles of guinea pigs. He reported in a paper given at a meeting of the Société de biologie in Paris that after injecting himself with the elixir, he needed less sleep, could stand for longer in his laboratory, ran up stairs, ate more, and had no trouble moving his bowels. Most thrilling was that the jet of his urine, low before his self-treatment, had afterward grown stronger and more arched.

Dr. Serge Voronoff, a Russian surgeon working in France, was the first to practice xenotransplantations. In 1917, funded by an American socialite whom he eventually married, Voronoff began grafting the testicles of young goats onto older ones. In 1920 he inserted slices of baboon testicles into a man's scrotum. He also transplanted the testicles of young executed criminals into elderly millionaires. He claimed this process raised sex drive, improved memory, and made reading glasses obsolete. Eventually he inserted monkey ovaries into women. This practice became so popular that, to keep up with the demand, he set up his own monkey farm on the Italian Riviera and hired a circus animal trainer to run it. Voronoff was so sought-after that in the 1920s, at the height of his fame, he took over the entire first floor of a Paris hotel with his chauffeur, butlers, personal assistants, and two mistresses.

These examples of remedies, hormonal and surgical, seemed far-fetched, the kind of witchy concoction sold by itinerant medicine men from the backs of wooden wagons, quacks who claimed magical results from elixirs made of lamb's blood and duck liver, until you learn that Premarin, the estrogen supplement taken by millions of women, is made from the urine of pregnant horses.

Introduced in 1942, Premarin remains popular today, with over nine million women taking the drug. An early ad in a medical journal shows a stylish gray-haired woman talking to two men at the theater. The caption reads "Help Keep Her This Way." After Dr. Wilson's *Feminine Forever* was published in 1966, prescriptions for Premarin soared to twenty-eight million by 1975. In the 1970s the drug was linked to uterine cancer. Wyeth Pharmaceuticals dropped the dosage and added progesterone, which was supposed to stop the drug from causing cancer.

———

Even as early as 1930, studies linked estrogen replacement to cancer in animals, but the drug company's message that hormones were natural, and that women needed them to stay balanced, was powerful to both doctors and aging women. Doctors began to push women, as they turned fifty, onto hormone therapy (HT). It was assumed, though no testing has ever backed it up, that estrogen protected against breast cancer, osteoporosis, and even heart disease. Many doctors, scientists, and husbands wanted women on HT. An ad from the late 1960s shows a photo of a harried bus driver: "He Suffers from Estrogen Deficiency." On the second page is a photo of an angry older female passenger: "She Is the Reason Why." In the 1970s, the singer Patti LaBelle touted HT in television commercials and the supermodel Lauren Hutton made talk show appearances, paid for by the drug company, to pitch hormone replacement therapy.

As late as 1998, companies used the image of a discombobulated woman to sell HT. In one ad, Picasso's *Weeping Woman* serves as the before image. The woman's face is smashed into swatches of green and yellow, and the teeth in her large horselike mouth are jagged. The after-HT image is of Renoir's *La loge*. The young, blue-eyed woman wears a black-and-white striped jacket. She has a pink rose in her hair and strings of pearls around her neck. She looks not only composed but also sexually available, with her loose bun, red lipstick, and pale rice-powder makeup. "No Other Estrogen Delivers Like

Estraderm," it reads—implying, of course, that HT will turn fragmented menopausal monsters into compliant fuckable girls.

In 2002, the Women's Health Initiative (WHI) study was stopped early because conditions that hormones were supposed to decrease—uterine and breast cancer, strokes, heart disease—all increased slightly when woman took hormone replacements. In 2005, the Radcliffe Institute for Advanced Studies held a conference where historians, scientists, feminists, and doctors came together to figure out what had gone wrong. Why, for more than fifty years, had doctors considered HT to be a magic bullet that protected women from age-related diseases? The most disturbing conclusion of the conference, and the one driven by an idea as old as the patriarchy itself, is that sex hormones explain women's behavior and so need to be controlled. "It is generally believed that women's nature and value derive from their capacity to bear children," the final report read, "and that it is in society's best interest to control women's reproductive systems."

Breast cancer continues to be linked with hormone therapy. A 2013 study reported that after the WHI findings, hormone use declined from 40 to 20 percent in the United States and breast cancer subsequently decreased as well: "A corresponding and substantial population-based decrease in breast cancer incidence was observed, particularly for estrogen receptor–positive breast cancers in women aged 50–69 years, which was attributed to decreased use of hormone therapy."

Hormone use remains a polarizing topic. Today, besides being made from horse urine, HT is also synthesized from soy and yam. Gels, patches, and creams exist in a variety of dosages. Women who have no family history of breast cancer or blood clotting can take HT for short periods of time to combat hot flashes and sleeplessness. Some continue to use HT to treat what they think of as a deficiency disease. Others feel hormones keep them from aging. All the personal accounts of menopause I found published in books ended with the come-to-Jesus moment of HT acceptance.

◎ ◎ ◎

Gayle Sand's 1993 *Is It Hot in Here or Is It Me?* registered the shock and suffering of menopause. But it cast this suffering as humorous. It's a spiky, uncomfortable, self-abasing kind of funny. Every night Sand rides her raging hormones like a "white water rafter on a Sealy Posturepedic." During hot flashes, she imagines herself as an ice cube, "but the ice always melts." Sex feels like a "root canal." Menopause has a magical effect on her sex life: "It makes it disappear." Her husband is cuckold, playing "second fiddle to a hot flash and a dry vagina." After trying alternative remedies, herbs, acupuncture, meditation, and yoga, Sand begins a full course of HT. Soon she is again feeling like her "old self."

The Silent Passage, Gail Sheehy's 1998 follow-up to her best-selling *Passages*, while less humorous than Sand's book, uses this same narrative trajectory of menopausal disorientation followed by HT salvation. "Won't I ever feel like me any-more?" Sheehy asks in her book's opening pages. I had this feeling in early menopause of disorientation, of loss of identity, one I also remember from the first months of menstruation. In adolescence, though I struggled, no one suggested I should block hormones to keep me as I was. Sheehy assumes that our reproductive phase is our only real phase, the healthy and valuable one, a period that should be held on to at all costs.

Christa D'Souza's book *Hot Topic* came out in 2016, well after the 2002 WHI study. While she offers a few positive examples of the menopausal transition—that hot flashes may aid life expectancy by making the brain more flexible and that menopause is a time to take stock of spiritual as well as physical changes—D'Souza, as a magazine editor and a fashionista, is clearly fearful of losing her femininity. She tells us in her preface that if we, her readers, don't take HT and "want to be butch" about menopause, she hopes we'll make it out the other side. After her search through alternative therapies and consultations with pro–hormone therapy doctors, she decides, even though she's had breast cancer, to stay on HT.

As Dr. Erika Schwartz, an internist in New York City, tells her, her worth outside the procreative hormonal years is zero. "Once you lose your hormones," Schwartz says, "you are nothing more than roadkill."

Saddest of the HT apologists is Suzanne Somers, who played Chrissy in the 1970s sitcom *Three's Company* and went on to sell everything from vitamins to the ThighMaster and Face-Master. Women like Somers who have spent their lives as sex symbols, making adaptations to male requirements, will share the negative view that men take of menopause. Men, Somers tells us in the first pages of *The Sexy Years*, find menopause "icky." What she calls the seven dwarfs of menopause, "Itchy, Bitchy, Sleepy, Sweaty, Bloated, Forgetful and All Dried Up," make women unlovable, even repulsive. Somers's book is similar to Dr. Wilson's *Feminine Forever* in its insistence on menopause as a negative passage, cured only by hormones. "Women who are afraid or confused about hormones will unfortunately experience the negative consequences of not taking them," Somers writes. "How about rotting bones, dried up vaginal tissue, droopy breasts, skin with no elasticity."

Somers pushes her readers to take hormones for the health benefits but also so that they remain compliant. "When estrogen levels sink during menopause," she writes, "a woman's body releases more testosterone, which causes women to be aggressive, but without that soft, clear-thinking, patient component to balance the aggression." This statement is both scientifically ungrounded and insidious. Somers wants women to take hormones so they remain feminine, kittenish purveyors of "horny sex." One of the gynecologists interviewed in the book, Dr. Uzzi Reiss, tells Somers that there are three types of women: twiggy, athletic, and curvy. The curvy type, he says, are short with D-cup breasts and weak muscles. They have extremely high estrogen. "I don't want to generalize but woman of this type (Curvy) are happier and less complex and it seems that their approach to sexuality is much simpler."

If we don't go on hormones, Somers tell us, our husbands are bound to leave us—much as how Dr. Wilson sympathizes with men who leave their "unhormonized masculine" wives. Somers repeats a half dozen times throughout *The Sexy Years* that menopausal women are "bitchy" and "impossible" to live with: "We can't sleep, we're hot and then cold, we're tired all the time, we break out in embarrassing sweats, we're bitchy, and we lose our sex drive, so after a while a man is going to say 'who needs this?' and go out and find the new, improved version of you." The antidote to this dilemma, according to Somers, is bioidentical hormones. Women must take them to remain young and lovable. She writes, "Finding balance for me has been like finding the fountain of youth." Somers advises as menopause begins going on hormones in dosages that replicate your body's chemistry at thirty and menstruating monthly until you die.

————

Long after I finished reading these books, they irritated me. At first I thought it was because each author goes on HT, a choice I saw as potentially dangerous unless you've had a hysterectomy. Maybe I was jealous. If my mother hadn't had breast cancer, if I didn't remember the smell of her mastectomy wound, the black threads stitched into her chest, I might have tried HT myself. Links between estrogen and cancer, while conclusive, are also percentage-wise relatively slight. Who am I to judge if a woman wants to take the risk?

It wasn't so much the hormones, I eventually realized, as the tone. Each book is the literary equivalent of a submissive dog offering its jugular to the more powerful species: man. In complete thrall to the culturally supported variety of moist, compliant femininity, these authors are unwilling to rethink youthful constructions of physicality and creativity or to accept responsibility for growth across the life span at every transitional phase. They pretend to break silences and offer revolutionary truths but in reality are spreading propaganda for the singularity and importance of the reproductive years and for estrogen replacement itself. They are like the girl in junior high who sees you floundering, but instead of supporting your otherness, shows you how to put on makeup, curl your hair, and diet so that you too can enter into a rigid femininity and join the generic popular crowd.

◎ ◎ ◎

Men have been marketed a similar, if less invasive, antiaging wonder drug in Viagra. It encourages men to deny their vulnerability, to resist the idea of aging and insist on penetrative sex over a lifetime. Older men are dealing with their own physical challenges and insecurities. Ads for Viagra play on their fears of not being able to get it up, of not pleasing the women in their lives. Counter to the message in the ads, many of the women I spoke to felt hostile toward the little blue pill. A friend told me that in the 1990s, she and her husband, then both in their sixties, had not had penetrative sex for years. Their sex life had grown so much better, "tender and adventurous." With the advent of Viagra, foreplay vanished. She felt forced, whenever he told her he had taken a pill, into having intercourse. "My husband was more interested in the idea of himself with an erection than he was in our actual sex life," she said. Men's obsession with penetration is understandable. Without intercourse the human race would not exist. But outside the procreation of children, men later in life would be wise to open up their idea of what constitutes a sexual act. Eventually my friend's husband figured out that a hard penis did not always lead to good sex. Other men may also come to this conclusion. "The bedroom may be the place where the Viagra myth ends," writes Meika Loe in her book *The Rise of Viagra*. "To [the drugmaker] Pfizer's horror, while millions of men asked their doctors for a prescription . . . only half requested a refill."

● ● ●

After I stopped cycling, I was able to feel both the wonder of cycling and its relentlessness. As a teenager, I thought of my ovaries as baskets full of eggs. In actuality the ovaries are less baskets and more high-tech superlabs. Eggs are maintained at a variety of stages. Fluid-filled blisters called follicles, each containing one egg, are basted with hormones. Female eggs are the biggest cell in a woman's body, about the size of a grain of sand and twenty-six times bigger than a blood cell. After eggs receive a signal to begin the process of maturation, it takes about 150 days before they are released. Egg cells have a different embryological origin than every other tissue of the body. They are also potentially immortal and supersensitive and have an inner intelligence. Scientists believe that the huge number of eggs that at first develop inside a female fetus's ovaries—nearly seven million—is a vestige from when we were fish spraying out eggs on the ocean floor.

The ripening egg, once chosen, is responsible for the variety of hormonal changes across the menstrual cycle. Each day of the month, a woman's hormonal balance is slightly different, which means a woman's brain chemistry is different every day. In the last days before menstruation, when progesterone drops, the brain is 25 percent different chemically than it is a day earlier in the cycle. Recent brain research suggests that the female brain is so deeply affected by hormones that the increase or decrease affects a woman's reality. For a cycling woman, the days just before her period, when hormones drop, are most like the hormonal landscape of menopause. What the culture ridicules as PMS—saying it stands for *pass my shotgun*, *psychotic mood shift*, or *pimples may surface*; joking that "they call it *PMS* because *mad cow disease* was already taken"—I remember as a time flooded with a delicate longing, a soul sickness, a sense of sudden lucidity.

"Cycling," one woman told me, "I felt like there was a stranger in my body." Many echo this feeling of a lack of control. "I move this body around," writes Samantha Irby in her essay "Hysterical!," "but I am not actually in charge of it." Another woman feels her body while cycling was "constantly betraying me." During her periods, another woman felt like "a big heavy mammal." Her pain was brutal. "I felt like I was giving birth to an alien," she said. Another remembers her periods being like six-day lava eruptions: "I'd jump out of my bed and blood spread everywhere. It was like a crime scene." Many women can't believe, after cycling, what they had to endure. "It's almost like the hormones made me feel dirty. It was like cancer—they took over my body each month," one said. Older women are incredulous when looking back: "Was that really me? Did I really go through all that?" and "It seems unimaginable now what I suffered. Did I really have to fool with bleeding every month for forty years?"

Once the hormonal onslaught is over, its beginnings can also seem surreal, freakish. One woman remembered the terrifying feelings stoked by hormones morphing her from girl to woman. "Sprouting breasts, hips, acne, my body had already (at 11) begun to feel unfamiliar—painful beginnings of breasts disturbed my flat chest, black hairs appeared like thin sprouts under my armpits." Another woman remembered her early girlhood receding: "When I looked in the bedroom mirror, I wondered, Who is this person?"

My daughter, too, felt the incredulity, the otherness of menstruating. When she was nine, I explained about the hormones, the egg, the uterus, the blood. In health class she learned the biology of the cycle, though she was more fascinated and disturbed by the slide show of genitalia infected with various venereal diseases. Each year I'd give her a refresher. She was going to bleed, but she wasn't wounded. It was natural. She was thirteen when I picked her up from the subway station and she announced that it had happened. During her oral report on Oedipus in English class, she felt a warm sensation between her legs. I gave her the heating pad and Advil and reminded her of the stash of tampons and sanitary napkins under the bathroom sink.

The next month, I was in my office when she burst in, her face fearful. "I got it again!" I realized then how abstract all my explanations had been, how inconceivable. I explained that, yes, she'd menstruate every month. "I thought you *got* your period," she said, "and that was *it*." She seemed dazed while I explained again. The egg, the uterus, the hormones, the sloughing off, the blood. "You mean every month I'm going to bleed?" I nodded. Her reaction reminded me of how unfathomable all female transitions—menstruation, birth, menopause—actually are. Our bodies shape-shift and writhe. What my daughter said next registered her shock but also that she'd absorbed at least a little of my family's Christianity: "Goddamn you, Jesus!"

◉ ◉ ◉

The only side effect of a lack of hormones that actively worries me is declining brainpower. Dr. Julie Dumas, a neurobiologist at the University of Vermont, did a study in which she tested the memories of menopausal women who complained of fuzzy thinking against those of non-complaining women. She found that not only was there no difference between the two groups but that the complainers did a little better on memory tests than the non-complainers. "Frankly," Dumas told me, "the studies are all over the place because cognition isn't only biological; there is also experience, emotion, the richer stuff that menopause does not alter."

Some studies do find that older women are slower on cognitive tests. When parsed, though, many of these studies also hint at the steadiness of the menopausal brain. Dr. Benicoo Frey of the Women's Health Clinic in Ontario, Canada, wanted to see if menopausal women had slower mental eflexes than fertile women. In 2008 he tested both groups. He used photographs with either happy or fearful faces, with the words "happy" or "fear" written in red over the eyes. Some of the photos were mislabeled, and women had to press a button when the word-face matchup was off. Dr. Frey found that in the first trial both groups scored equally, but in subsequent trials the younger group scored slightly better. What interests me is not this discrepancy but that the MRIs of the older women showed less activity in the amygdala, a part of the brain that registers emotion. This could mean either that the older women were less afraid of the fearful faces or that the slight delay was not slow but Zen-like, mindful. "We hypothesized," Dr. Frey told me, "that the midlife transition might be associated with a shift toward greater top-down regulation with subsequent more cognitive control and less emotional reactivity." In other words, menopausal women, counter to cultural stereotypes, react with fewer emotional highs and lows than younger women, and they pause to contemplate before they answer.

◎ ◎ ◎

The Sisters of Perpetual Adoration are a Carmelite order of eleven menopausal nuns who live in the Haight-Ashbury section of San Francisco. The order, originally established in Guadalajara, Mexico, moved because of religious persecution to California in 1928. The nuns wear white tunics, red scapulars, and black habits. Their main occupation is prayer, and they pray throughout the day both separately and to-gether. Twice a month they pray for twenty-four hours straight. All life is subsumed in prayer, and even the nun's hot flashes are considered spiritual. "I think of it as getting closer to God," Sister Betty told a researcher, "of getting closer to eternity." The neuroscientist Dr. Sohila Zadran, of Igantia Therapeutics, is working with the sisters to see if hot flashes may protect the brain and be one of the reasons why women tend to live longer than men. Zadran believes flashes are an example of an active Darwinian adaptation. She told me about the "halo effect," in which the nuns seem to catch flashes from one another. By setting up an infrared camera in the convent chapel, Zadran saw for herself the halo effect. First one nun started to glow as the camera registered heated blood flooding into her arms and legs, and then one after another, a red aura flared up around each nun's body. "It was an eerie sight," Dr. Zadran told me, "the glowing nuns and behind them the glowing stained-glass windows."

The Holy Spirit again. Though this time in a scientific frame. Inside a flash I often think of Mary at the first Pentecost. What Acts identifies as an "upper room" may have been sealed, warm, constricting. If Jesus was thirty-three when he died, Mary would have been in either perimenopause or menopause itself. Maybe she flashed first and the heat spread, like it did among the nuns, from disciple to disciple. "To be a created thing is not necessarily to be afflicted," Simone Weil writes, "but it is necessary to be exposed to affliction."

We are promised many things if we go on HT: level moods; sleep; smooth skin; wet, pliable pussies. But what do we gain by not going on hormones, by going through the junkie-like withdrawal, staying with this disorienting and relentless adaptation? Darwinian adaptations are glacially slow, impossible to monitor. They occur through gradual modification of existing structures. Over thousands of years a male bird gets bluer feathers to help him attract a mate, and a dolphin's hoofs slowly spread into fleshy flippers. My withdrawal is adaptive as well as liminal. De Quincey claimed that the agony of his withdrawal from opium felt more like a birth than a death: "During the whole period of diminishing the opium I had the torments of a man passing out of one mode of existence into another."

◎ ◎ ◎

In "Choosing Paradise," a story by the British writer Sara Maitland, an aged Eve sits on the stone wall that surrounds the Garden of Eden. She's found the garden again but she's torn about going back. She remembers her youthful happiness there but also doesn't want to desert the life she's made for herself. Eve decides against reentering perfection. She does not tell Adam she's found the garden again—or that she's stopped menstruating: "The curse is lifted, he does not rule me anymore." Rather than claw back what she's lost and remain in perpetual stasis, Eve decides to go with acceleration. In choosing her aging body, her imperfect life, Eve makes a decision that many women do in refusing HT. "I realize looking back how controlled I was by my hormones," one woman told me. "It's a relief to no longer be driven by them." Eve's decision links back to her first curiosity-driven bite. "Going forward," she reminds us, "is more interesting than being happy."

5 ● Demigirl in Kemmering

Without hormones my femininity is fraying. Twice I've been called "sir." Once by a parking lot attendant and a second time by the young man who bagged my groceries. I did not correct them. Instead I tried to sit with the idea I'd been misgendered. I don't possess the strong female signifiers I once did. My hair is not long and shiny, my skin is no longer smooth. Plus I do less to support my gender artificially. I wear more androgynous clothing and rarely put on makeup. I've lost interest in *doing* my female gender, propping it up. When I do dress up for a wedding or a bat mitzvah, I feel like a drag queen, performing a gender out of sync with my physicality; but unlike a drag queen, I don't feel that gender is natural or correct.

What is this femininity that lack of estrogen is letting me slip out from under, as if I were stripping off a pair of tight pants? Freud felt femininity to be mysterious: "We must conclude that what constitutes masculinity and femininity is an unknown characteristic which anatomy alone cannot lay hold of." Femininity for Freud was a riddle of nature. He felt that the prepubescent girl was a bisexual creature: "An individual is not a man or a woman but always both." Freud believed that femininity is always fragile; it hung in the balance not only in girlhood but after: "In the course of a woman's life there is a repeated alteration between periods in which masculinity or femininity gain the upper hand." He even explained that men's confusion about women was because of our inherent androgyny: "'The enigma of women' may perhaps be derived from this expression of bisexuality in women's lives."

As his lecture ended, Freud expressed difficulty in treating women. He felt it was harder for them to change than it was for men: "It is as though, indeed, the difficult development to femininity had exhausted the possibilities of the person concerned." I'd argue that it is not an early individuation that exhausts women but instead the continual stress of maintaining and holding up our femininity.

Virginie Despentes, in her 2010 manifesto *King Kong Theory*, is unashamed of not wanting to be feminine. She does not care that she is not a "hot sexy number." But, she explains, she is "livid that—as a girl who does not attract men—I am constantly made to feel as if I shouldn't even be around." Rather than work to reestablish her femininity, she's relieved to let it go. "Never before has a society demanded as much proof of submission to an aesthetic ideal, or as much body modification, to achieve physical femininity." She points out that it's not that some women are feminine failures, but that femininity itself is not a reliable goal.

I came of age in Virginia, in a feminizing culture where the male/female binary was brutally enforced. I rose at 6:00 a.m. to wash, blow-dry, hot-curl, and hair-spray my hair every single day. If I missed a day, I could be accused of being a greasy-haired freak. I was often whispered about and laughed at for making mistakes at performing my gender. I was always at the edge of popularity, barely holding on, and my femininity was under constant surveillance. Girls who were supposedly my friends criticized my hair, the way I walked, the smear of foundation on my chin, the black stubble under my arms. And, if I am honest, I shamed girls below me on the popularity ladder. Femininity was rigid, and any attempt to get out of the cage led to ridicule.

There was a girl in my high school who embodied the perfect feminine ideal. Amy was so thin that boys often swept her up and carried her in one arm like a doll. Her thinness now reads as anorexia, but then it was miraculous. In her pink gauze shirts and white painter pants she was a sprite, her lay-ered hair perfect against her small head. Though she must have spoken, I can't remember Amy ever saying anything. It was as if she was too feminine to even communicate. Talk-ing would have weighted her perfect lightness. At parties, it was not unusual for boys to fight over Amy. Her delicateness drove them insane. And her emotional volatility was hon-ored. "She cries," one boy told me with admiration, "if you say anything to her at all."

Earlier, as a little girl of eight, I'd take a magazine picture of a Chinese woman's tiny destroyed feet from where I kept it inside the pages of a book and spread it out on my bed. The photo showed toes pushed underneath, the arches broken so that the heel and pad compressed. The feet looked like man-gled cat paws, the fleshy claws of a small mythic beast. I wor-shipped the tiny lotus feet, not sexually as Chinese men had but with a pervert's thrill for the anguish and hobbling that lay ahead.

● ● ●

Defeminization is not on the list of menopausal symptoms. Even if ungendering were listed, it would be framed as nega-tive rather than as the rare opportunity it is to finally slip outside the brutal binary system. While a few of the women I interviewed felt, in and after menopause, even more like women, most felt a gender shift. For some, like my high school friend, this was a defeat: "I feel like a washed-up version of my former self now that I've lost all my female attributes."

Trans women who stop or lessen hormone therapy can also experience menopausal-like symptoms. The science fiction writer Rachel Pollack has found, as she ages, that the outer world is more open to her variety of femininity. She *passes* more often than she did as a younger woman: "In my early life store clerks and waiters were uncertain as to what to call me, miss or sir." Getting older seems to have changed that. "Maybe it's just the way society regards older women. The bonds of femininity loosen a little."

Some women, like my high school friend, feel that the loss of femininity diminishes their value; others, like Rachel, have found unanticipated benefits. Gender slippage can be invigorating. "I do feel between the sexes and I love it." Another woman told me she no longer feels like a woman or a man: "I am between, but this has given me unexpected confidence." One woman told me she'd always considered herself on the androgynous spectrum. "With reduced estrogen I feel even less feminine, and frankly I'm good with that."

In menopause, femininity strains, splits at the seams, and what once seemed natural now has to be constructed, as Judith Butler explains in her influential 1990 book *Gender Trouble*, like "so many styles of the flesh." Butler writes that gender is not stable. "Rather, gender is an identity tenuously constructed in time, instituted in an exterior space through a *stylized repetition of acts*."

Sometimes within a flash I feel as if my femininity is not figuratively but actually physically coming apart, being slowly but continuously burned off. It is often by heat that physical matter is transformed. I feel less like a woman or, at the very least, less like the woman I was. Someone who at book parties worked harder to introduce men to one another than to express myself, who often used my corporeal form, rather than my brain, for first effect.

Even in my teen years, when I was most feminine, both physically and in performance, I often longed to get out from under the strict Southern definition of femininity. I'd fantasize that I was forced into the shower fully clothed. The narrative was always the same: my dress and hose got drenched, and I peeled them off, as well as my bra and underwear. Warm water washed away my makeup, the pancake base, the blush, the mascara, and eye shadow. My curled and sprayed hair was flattened against my head. Sometimes a pair of old-fashioned black-handled scissors hung on a hook in the shower, and I'd cut my hair. Dark wet clumps around the drain like animal fur. When I came out—and this is the part that was nearly orgasmic in its pleasure—I saw in the mirror that I was no longer so tightly female. I didn't look like a boy either, as I had breasts. I was in the middle.

I feel drawn in menopause—as I transition, as my estrogen lessens—to people who are also experiencing an ungendering. I want to read stories not of propped-up femininity but of people who are disoriented but also electrified by their new hormonal configuration.

◉ ◉ ◉

When people talk about menopausal bodies, they are often cruel. There are the base names: *dried-up cunt, old hag*. Some doctors peddling hormonal solutions, like Wilson and Schwartz, have called us *castrates, neuters, roadkill*. Websites list off endless symptoms phrased in the meanest way possible: sagging skin, atrophied vagina, senile ovaries. The lists are both intimate and cold, like a scientist's field notes on an aging, captive animal. It's important to be honest about the symptoms. Hiding them does no good. I am not blind. I can see that I have a tummy, heavier thighs, gray strands in my pubic hair. The lines around my mouth are deeper, the dark circles under my eyes, which used to appear only when I was exhausted, now seem to be permanent. I look always a little burnt-out, a little feral. I want honesty. But the endless negative lists don't help me, don't lift me up. "The female body is marked within the masculine discourse," Simone de Beauvoir writes, "whereby the masculine body, in its conflation with the universe, remains unmarked."

At times I feel another body slipping out from my original one. Once when coming up from the subway, I saw a reflection of an older man in a bodega window. I stared for a few seconds before I realized it was me. Other times I will see a neck crinkled like crepe paper in the car's rearview mirror, or a white and chalky foot, and be unable for several seconds to connect the flesh to my own.

This sensation is alienating but also oddly thrilling. For decades I've tried, mostly unsuccessfully, to get out of the way so the force of the universe could use me as a conduit. Only recently, with the onset of menopause and the breakdown of my former identity, do I finally feel I am making a little progress. "It is fundamental not to recognize oneself," the French critic Paul B. Preciado writes in his book *Testo Junkie*. "Derecognition, disidentification is a condition for the emergence of the political as the possibility of transforming reality."

Several years ago I heard the transgender musician Anohni, who at the time used male pronouns and went by 'Antony Hegarty,' talking to Terry Gross on *Fresh Air*. When Gross asked if she planned to "surgically alter [herself]," Anohni was frustrated. "Something very reductive tends to occur when discussing transgender people. Society wants to reduce them in a crude way. There is an obsession with their sexuality, even their genital configuration."

Sound familiar? Are our ovaries senile, our vaginas dry, our libidos broken? "There is a cruelty in that," Anohni went on, insisting that being transgender is a condition of the spirit. "Transgender people," she argued, and I would add menopausal women as well, "have different spirits." They should not be boxed in and defined solely by their physicality. "Trans people have a lot of potential," Anohni said, "a potential which often remains unacknowledged and even unexplored, because individuals fall victim to society's impression of them. Society reduces them."

◎ ◎ ◎

I track the mental and physical metamorphosis of my hormonal withdrawal while reading testaments by transitioning men and woman. These books posit hormonal change as both arduous and interesting. The British writer Juliet Jacques doesn't believe in the traditional redemptive trans story; she feels her experience with gender reassignment was more like "jumping through a bunch of hoops while working boring jobs." Given Estelle, the same drug used for menopausal symptoms, Jacques notices her skin begin to soften, her hair getting thicker. Her feelings are harder to ignore. She is more relaxed and cries more easily. During her transition she feels in a "position between male and female."

In *Whipping Girl,* Julia Serano also reports that on estrogen she cries more easily and can't stop crying once she starts. She feels during her transition "an ungendering, an unraveling." She grasps how close men and women are. "I have found that women and men are not separated by an insurmountable chasm, as many people believe. Actually most of us are only a hormone prescription away from being perceived as the opposite sex."

Max Wolf Valerio writes in his book *The Testosterone Files* about his transition from punk rock, bohemian, lesbian feminist to heterosexual man. He describes what he goes through as "a unique intensive fire." He is making an "erotically charged boundary crossing." He claims changing sexes is "an adventure, an investigation and an opportunity to live beyond the given and the commonplace." He even goes so far as to compare the mental state of his transition to menopause: "A woman I know going through menopause reports that she too feels this clarity and sometimes feels like a wise old owl who can see for a very long distance."

Before his transition, when he had more estrogen, Valerio felt that every object had an emotional weight, a gravity that pulled feeling into it. "The world had an intensity of feeling, tender, sentimental, subtle, deep. Everything around me was soaked in these feelings." On estrogen, he felt "submerged in a sweet dense fog, like walking through liquid—slow, languid."

On testosterone, Valerio describes having feelings similar to those of women undergoing the menopausal transition. He is more emotionally self-sufficient, more independent. One woman, outside of cycling, told me, "Now my mind is much freer to work on my own ideas without those hormones haunting the house." Valerio feels energetic, cranked up. He is often sleepless, space has "crystalized," and he moves in a "staggering space of emotional equilibrium. Estrogen had a soporific effect, dreamy, nearly beatific." Now everything appears more three-dimensional, lines are sharply drawn, and visual perception enlarges.

Anger is also easier to access. Valerio feels and acts out his anger, and for the first time in his life he is better able to stand up for himself. I also feel angry more often, a menopausal condition that doctors classify as hormonal irritability but that I'm starting to see as a gateway to authenticity. "One of the most predictable outcomes of female-to-male transition," Valerio writes, "is an increase in intolerance for bad behavior from others."

As Valerio comes through his transition, he continues to bind his chest. His voice has deepened, and he has facial hair, but it's emotionally that he most feels the change. The emotions that the objects of his life had accrued are now faint.

"Everything is flatter, flatter and brighter, as though a fog has lifted. I'm not depressed. There's a freedom, a bright clarity."

During menopause I slip out from under a claustrophobic femininity. But I also don't feel fully masculine. I feel in the middle, a third gender. They. At the Twitter account recommended to me by my agender student Elliot, @askabinary, I find feelings and questions I very much identify with.
—I think a lot more like a boy than a girl but I don't think I want to stick with one gender.
—I am sure I am non-binary but I pretend to be a cis female in public and though it sometimes annoys me, I don't really intend to change that view.
—I identify as demigirl but there are times when I fluctuate from agender to demigirl to female. Can I still identify as demigirl instead of gender flux?

When I meet Elliot, who has recently moved from *she* to *they*, for lunch, they tell me they are sick of chest binding and will soon have top surgery. Elliot has short black hair and dresses with impish androgyny in men's pants and band T-shirts. They feel that once their chest is smooth and light, they will be more likely to wear dresses. Elliot now understands that their anorexia in high school was not to make them thin and feminine but an attempt to be light, unburdened, more like a boy but also between sexes. "Female," they tell me, "has always felt like an itchy sweater."

———

Riding the Q train I look around at my fellow passengers, telling myself that I shouldn't gender them as male or female. I try to experience each person as their own unique self. "Being a drag king," Preciado writes in *Testo Junkie*, "is seeing through the matrix of gender, noticing that men and women are performative and somatic fictions, convinced of their material reality." Or as my twenty-two-year-old daughter, Abbie, patiently explains when I tell her I think there should be ten or twenty genders: "You don't get it. Each person is their own gender. There are as many genders as there are human beings." On the subway, a few riders stick to the opposite ends of the binary: a woman in tight jeans, a full face of makeup, carefully coiffed hair; and two men sitting with their legs spread, biceps stretching out from under the sleeves of their T-shirts. Everyone else is more in the middle. An older Chinese lady in sneakers, khakis, and a sweatshirt, her hair cut close to her head. A heavyset guy with man breasts grading math papers. It seems that there is both absentminded and intentional androgyny: a young woman in big Clark Kent glasses, a white button-down, and men's pants; and a young Hispanic man in tight jeans, a glittery sweater, and big hoop earrings.

Aristophanes claimed that besides men and women, there was once a third sex, a creature who had four hands, four feet, and two heads. Male/female, female/female, and male/male, this creature was round and so strong that it often attacked the gods by rolling right up to Mount Olympus. So Zeus, hoping to diminish the third sex's power, decided to split them. Cut them like an "apple that is halved for pickling or as you might cut an egg in half with a hair."

I first heard about the beast with two backs in the sixth grade, when I'd just begun to be lonely in my childhood bed, feeling a desire not only for sex but also for a male counterpart. "Sliced in two like a flatfish," Aristophanes writes, "each of us is perpetually hunting for the matching half of himself." Now I wonder if I didn't misinterpret my adolescent longing for a separate male body. Maybe what I wanted all along was an inner return, a healing of male and female inside myself.

"The body . . . ," Michel Foucault writes, "is the heart of the world . . . from which all possible places, real or utopian, emerge and radiate."

◎ ◎ ◎

The last Sunday in August, after I drop my daughter, Abbie, at the bus station in Monticello, New York, to go back to college, I drive back up 17 and, at Roscoe, I turn in toward Crystal Lake. Abbie has been with me for a few days in the country before college starts. We tubed down the Delaware River, thrift-shopped in Callicoon, baked lemon cake. There is little tension between myself and my daughter. I attribute this mostly to her temperament. Even as a little girl, when she got frustrated with me, she'd hold my big hand in her tiny one and say, "You didn't understand. Let me explain."

It also helps that I did not foist a fixed femininity on her. I dressed her mostly like a tomboy and never told her she looked like a princess. I tried hard not to model female shame. I never told her to eat like a lady. When she went out in cut-offs and ripped tights, the uniform of high school girls in her era, I didn't say she looked slutty. I never mentioned her weight. I never told her, as my own mother told me, to wrap my bloody tampon in twenty layers of toilet paper and hide it at the bottom of the bathroom waste bin. At one point over the weekend, Abbie asked me if I knew that some boys were grossed out by menstrual blood. I loved both her surprise and her indignation. Yes, I said. I knew this.

I drive down a long gravel road toward the lake. On either side ferns unfurl. Everything, even the light, is mossy green. I park and walk around to the far side of the lake, carrying my towel and my wet suit. There is, in my usual spot, a mother with her young daughter. They sit on a blanket near the lake's edge. The mother, her brown hair in a ponytail, is wearing a faded gingham bikini, and her tiny daughter, a Hello Kitty one-piece. Her bare arms and legs impossibly thin, she piles rocks and grass onto her mother's stomach. Her bangs are cut straight across her forehead, and her brown eyes show darts of silver. She drizzles the broken blades of grass over her mother's belly, laughing. As I pull on my wet suit, the little girl looks up and watches me push my hair under a bathing cap, adjust my goggles, wade in.

———

The water, while heated at the top, is cold deeper down. I dive under and stroke. Swimming in the lake is the only true remedy for my hormonal withdrawal. I don't flash in the cool water, and after a swim, I get a few flash-free hours. I stroke, my hands and mouth sending up bubbles that swirl to the surface. The water around me is green-gold and translucent. Below, gray-green and mysterious. Since I've stopped my struggle to be beautiful, I am overtaken by beauty more often. I stroke toward the sun so that rays splinter as they hit the water and seem to encase me, carry me as if I were a spaceship, lifted in my own radiating light.

My wet suit makes me buoyant, gives me grace and speed. I can pause, float without treading. I am weightless, light. Swimming, I feel the least confined by my femininity. I wonder if part of the work of life for everyone might be to synthesize the sexes. "When you make the two one," Jesus says in the Gnostic Gospel of Thomas, "when you make the inside like the outside, and the outside like the inside, and the upper like the lower and when you make male and female into a single one, then you will enter the kingdom."

The most surprising outcome of my ungendering has been that the male God I grew up with has lost his power. When I was a child, God was always and everywhere male. But the divine mystery cannot be domesticated into a fixed, petrified image. That's idolatry. My feeling less feminine means I no longer need a masculine God. I feel, instead, a new force, latent in the black expanse beneath me. There is nothing predictable or tame about this spirit. Elemental. Androgynous. Chaotic. Not found hovering ghostlike in nature, but the actual engine that drives nature. An atavistic force, the King Kong of Despentes's *King Kong Theory*, a pregendered wildness that we lose claim to when we enter the strict binary. *Tehom*, the Bible calls it: the deep.

I turn around. The sun glitters on the water in front of me, makes a path for me to follow back, sequin to sequin. "There is a kind of story, God," Fanny Howe writes, "that glides along under everything else that is happening, and this kind of story only jumps out into the light like a silver fish when it wants to see where it lives in relation to everything else."

The lake bottom comes slowly into focus. Ancient, moonlike, rounded rocks covered in soft sludge, then a zigzag of knobby tree roots. I put my feet down beside the muddy bank, and as I stretch up, water rushes out of my wet suit. The material that kept me light in the water is now soaked and heavy. I use both hands on the grassy edge to steady myself. The little girl runs up to watch. Her brown eyes are liquid, serious. She runs back to her mother, cups her small hand around her mother's ear, and whispers loudly enough for me to hear: *Let's ask her what she found.*

6 ● Lessons in Demonology

I walked up the Q train station steps, pushed through the turnstile, and headed out into the stormy fall night. Even as I left the station, anger swirled in my chest, severe and combustible. I moved away from the dark trees of Prospect Park down toward Flatbush Avenue. Some people say fury makes them blind, unable to see the world around them. I felt the opposite. Rage focused my attention. The wet asphalt reflected a red ATM sign. In the market on the corner, I watched a policeman buy a coffee in a white paper cup. Down Flatbush past the nail salon with the wall of multicolored polish, then past the vegetable stand, lemons and limes shining just inside the glass door, and left on Midwood, where I walked under wild trees, as different from trees in calm sunlight as a living person is from a zombie. Branches moved frantically in the greenish streetlight.

I had my worries. I wasn't sure I could get the money together for my daughter's college, and I'd developed a mysterious skin condition, with hives rising up under my bra strap and at the waist of my jeans. Those were on a back burner. In the forefront that night was a rage with a singular focus directed at my husband.

Mike has many great qualities, but neatness is not one of them. He often jokes about how, while he was away, a neighbor who glanced into his window assumed his house had been ransacked and called the police, how he caught a jar of peanut butter on fire, and how he lived for years with water leaking out of an overhead light fixture. When I visited him in Virginia while we were dating long-distance, a raccoon who had learned to use his cat door came nightly into the kitchen to go through the trash.

Mike moved to Brooklyn in 2005 and we got married in 2008. Our shared domesticity didn't change his slovenliness. He seemed to find his messiness charming, but to me, who had lived the ten years before as a struggling single mother, his lapses not only meant more work but also danger. My mother had died the year before, alone in her house in Albany, New York. By the time I drove up from Brooklyn, her body had been removed, but my brothers and I found her house in shambles, newspapers all over the floor, drawers tipped out, empty food containers scattered everywhere.

Mike's messiness, to me, was tinged with death, sinister. I was afraid his carelessness would eventually somehow hurt me and my daughter. He left his dirty clothes everywhere, left drawers and cabinets open in the kitchen, and he never offered to cook meals, change the kitty litter, or make the bed.

In hindsight I can see that what I was actually mad about went much deeper than Mike's messiness. I'd lived alone with my daughter for ten years, and I'd forgotten how easy it is for men to focus. To be all-consumed with their work, their sports teams, their computers. I was as angry at him for making me bear the brunt of our shared domestic duties as I was at myself for feeling weighted by and responsible for them.

What marked this night as different, though, is how hard I struggled with conflicting forces inside myself. Should I confront him or should I continue to stuff it? As I turned onto Bedford, I knew there would be dishes in the sink, that the bed would not be made. I'd find his underwear on the floor, his spit in the bathroom sink, even his pee in the toilet. Cold wind drove tiny bits of ice against my face. Dog shit and chicken bones littered the sidewalk, and the red stoplight swung around like a gigantic demonic charm. I felt as if the wind moved not only against my jacket, flattening out the down, but also through my skull, blasting open the door between me and my rage.

◎ ◎ ◎

Like many women, I got sad, not angry, for most of my pre-menopausal life. I pushed down and compressed my anger until I could almost convince myself it did not exist. I reveled in being split, diaphanous. It was a little like being high, having no singular self. Being weightless, like a ghost. "In order to avoid her rage," writes the therapist Mary Valentis, "a woman may have to numb herself to all feeling."

◎ ◎ ◎

In her 2004 *Anger Workbook for Women*, Dr. Laura Petracek uses worksheets and exercises to apply cognitive behavioral techniques to help angry women. She stresses in the foreword how uncomfortable the culture is in general with female anger, how women are told anger is not ladylike, how our anger is defeminizing, even dehumanizing. Angry women are so threatening that they've been accused of being demonically possessed. Angry men are just men. Angry women are stigmatized and stereotyped: shrill wife, crazy ex-girlfriend, feminazi. I recognize myself in the details of women who are so afraid of their anger that they control not only its expression but also their awareness of its existence.

I felt affinity with the ideas in the *Anger Workbook* as well as with the ghost trapped inside its pages. In pencil, the book's former owner had checked off symptoms that had developed because of her own tamped-down rage. Frightening thoughts. Ironic humor. Smiling while hurting. Disturbing dreams.

Slowing down movement. Suddenly refusing eye contact with another person. Laughing when nothing funny is going on.

As a young woman, I was drawn to female characters whose repressed anger fermented into a melancholy that made them feel unreal, ghostly. In Jean Rhys's novel *Good Morning, Midnight*, Sasha Jansen stares through a storefront window at an older woman, an aged version of herself, trying on a hat. The woman's expression is *terrible, hungry, despairing, hopeful*. "At any moment you expected her to start laughing the laugh of the mad." Sasha, whose husband left her after their baby died, lives in Paris, dreaming of a well-lit room with a private bath, instead of the dingy room in a cheap hotel she shares with another ghost, a man who seems to be always standing in his white bathrobe on the landing.

Embarrassed by her shabby clothes, as well as the barren body underneath, Sasha longs to be invisible. She understands invisibility to be a mental state: "You must make your mind vacant, neutral, then your face also becomes vacant, neutral—you are invisible." As the novel ends, Sasha is so unhappy that a part of her, phantomlike, splits off. "Who is this crying? The same one who laughed on the landing, kissed him, and was happy. This is me, this is myself, who is crying. The other," Rhys writes, "how do I know who the other is? She isn't me."

Lonely people, a 2007 study found, are more likely to believe in the supernatural. This is linked to the greater fear people who live alone have of home invasions. If you don't have real friends, the mind makes up ghostly malevolent ones. I was at my loneliest the year I was writer in residence at Ole Miss, in Oxford, living in a stately home across from Faulkner's home Rowan Oak. My first marriage was on the rocks and I was facing a future as a single mother. One night after I had put my daughter into her crib, I was in my bed reading. The large room was dark, with only the cone of inverted light illuminating the pages of my book. The master bedroom was as big as my entire Brooklyn apartment. Outside I heard wind chimes in my neighbors' yard and branches from the dogwood scratching against the house.

The Victorian writer Cynthia Asquith, in her story "God Grant That She Lye Still," tells of a woman so permeable that the spirit of a dead girl infiltrates her body and eventually her mind. "I don't know how to explain," she tells her doctor, "but what I mean is that there is no real permanent essential Me." Asquith herself wrote about having this sensation: "I feel so hopelessly fluid. So indefinite. A different person with whichever friend I'm with and no one at all when I'm by myself." Asquith felt herself to be a ghost. In her stories living and dead characters find themselves interchangeable. "I believe . . . ," the critic Ruth D. Weston writes, "that Asquith internalized a patriarchal perception so self-contradictory as to defy rational explanation." The actual chill of "God Grant

That She Lye Still" is less the struggle the human narrator has with the ghost from a nearby graveyard, and more that, alone, Asquith feels "like water released from a broken bowl—something just spilling away—to be absorbed back into nothingness."

"Feeling of Presence has specific characteristics," says the science writer Rick Paulas in his essay "The Neuroscience of Ghosts." "If the patient was standing, the presence was felt as standing. If the patient was lying down, the patient felt as if the presence was lying down." During these episodes, three areas of the cerebral cortex light up, ones that deal with visual memory and perception. "These areas," Paulas writes, "give you the [feeling] that you are a specific body." If there are lesions in the brain, or if the brain is traumatized or stressed, it makes the assumption that someone else is in the room with you. There is a sort of doubling in the patient's body.

In Mississippi, I could keep it together during daylight hours, but at night a strange feeling of uncontainment came over me, as if I were bifurcating like the multiple images in a dressing-room mirror, splitting up into a multitude of selves. I had the sensation, as I sat up in my bed reading, that I was also sitting across the room reading. When I twisted the neck of my reading lamp, it illuminated the empty velvet love seat. Still, I felt a presence, a woman with my same weight and focus, but she wasn't melancholy like me. No. She was furious.

Many female ghosts are ineffectual. Like depressed people, they float around the house, miserable but unable to act. Others, though, have angry agency. Women in books and movies often make better ghosts than men; in a male-dominated society, their rights are repressed, and they are less likely to find justice in the material world. Female ghosts who were unhappy or victimized while alive can seek revenge after they enter the spirit world.

Bloody Mary is one such spirit. Both my mother and grandmother told me how, as girls, they along with their friends had tried to summon Bloody Mary. Abbie, my daughter, came home once spooked from a sleepover, telling me she and her best friend, Ginger, had seen a bloody woman in the mirror. The ritual varies according to decade and part of the country: Girls hold a hand mirror and walk up a flight of stairs backward chanting, "Bloody Mary." They flush the toilet and whirl around thirteen times. They prick their fingers, then smear the glass with blood. At slumber parties in the 1970s, my girlfriends and I turned off the bathroom light, lit a candle, and gathered around the mirror: "Where is your baby, Bloody Mary?"

Mary Tudor took the throne in 1553. She was nicknamed Bloody Mary for ordering three hundred of her subjects burned at the stake. This moniker seems unfair, considering her father, Henry VIII, put not only two of his wives but also fifty-seven thousand of his subjects to death. Being England's first female ruler, Mary Tudor was ridiculed and undermined. Her procreative struggles were mocked. Court doctors recorded that Mary suffered from heavy blood flow, pelvic pain, and cramps. At thirty-eight, she married Philip of Spain and soon after suffered a phantom pregnancy that led to a nervous breakdown. At forty-two, Mary had another phantom pregnancy. Some say she confused stomach cancer with a fetus, others that she had stopped menstruating because of menopause.

Begging a mirror for clues to the future, sometimes known as scrying, has a long history. Besides the Bloody Mary ritual and the evil queen's enchanted mirror in "Snow White," the practice appears in the Bible—"seeing through a glass darkly"—as well as in Chaucer, Spenser, and Shakespeare's *Macbeth*. The relationship, supernatural or not, between a woman and her mirror is complicated. Our reflection, day by day, reveals our abjectness. Menstruation sets off sexuality, and girls at this precipice are understandably anxious over what is to come, bodies bleeding monthly, opening up in childbirth, and eventually decaying with age. In Sylvia Plath's scrying poem, the mirror speaks: "Each morning it is her face that replaces the darkness. / In me she has drowned a young girl, and in me an old woman / Rises toward her day after day like a terrible fish."

◉ ◉ ◉

Fish, according to historians, were one of the few animals not suspected as a witch's familiar. Women could be accused of witchcraft for being too friendly with their cats. If a woman was seen talking to or looking at ferrets, hedgehogs, mice, rats, rabbits, squirrels, weasels, snakes, owls, or insects, then that woman was a witch. One witch supposedly kept bees under a rock and called them out so they could drink blood from her pricked finger.

Women in the sixteenth and seventeenth centuries, according to sources, could be accused of witchcraft if they begged at their neighbor's house for a pitcher of milk, if they crashed a wedding and asked for a sausage, if their plants were taller than their male neighbors', or if they were better at steering their ploughs than were their male neighbors. If, when a woman pulled a blanket down from a shelf, a toad jumped out, then she was a witch. If she was poor. Witch. If she was widowed. Witch. If she had neither father, son, husband, nor brother. Witch. If she was the midwife and, through no fault of her own, the baby died, she was a witch. If women appeared as witches in their neighbors' dreams, then they were witches. If they made herbal tinctures for sick neighbors, they were witches. If they regularly had black eyes, bruises on their arms or legs, and cuts over their bodies, then, as their husbands suggested, they'd been beaten by the devil and were definitely witches.

———

The most common clues for demonologists, though, were connected to menopause. Chin hairs. Witch. Wrinkles. Witch. Warts. Witch. If a woman had on her arm a skin tag, a bit of gray flesh that looked like a miniature teat, then she was a witch. If, in the presence of others, a woman grew red and perspired heavily, then she was a witch. If, in summer, unable to sleep, she wandered in her nightgown outside her house, then she was a witch. If she was quarrelsome, angry, spoke loudly, and moved, at times, in quick bursts of chaotic energy, to open a window or get a ladle of water, then she was definitely a witch.

In Ipswich, Massachusetts, in 1687, after her husband abandoned her, Rachel Clinton was forced to beg from house to house. She had not eaten in three days when she went to her neighbor Thomas Knowlton's house and asked his maid for meat and milk. When the maid denied her, Clinton pushed past her into the house. As Knowlton tried to remove her, she called him a hellhound, a whoremasterly rogue, and a limb of the devil. Just before he threw her out the door, Clinton looked directly into her neighbor's eyes and said she'd rather see the devil than him. Knowlton turned her in as a witch.

The devil in Sylvia Townsend Warner's 1926 novel, *Lolly Willowes*, is more understanding than any man. He both acknowledges Lolly's inner darkness—"I will give you the dangerous black night to stretch your wings in"—and her need for freedom. The book features Lolly, a fortysomething spinster who longs for autonomy and a deeper connection to nature. "One doesn't become a witch," Warner writes, "to run around being harmful, or to run around being helpful either . . . it's to escape all that . . . to have a life of one's own." As the novel ends, after meeting the devil, who looks like a gentle gamekeeper, Lolly feels giddy, as though she had been thrown into the air and *suddenly begun to fly.*

Alex Mar, the author of the 2016 memoir *Witches of America*, takes part in a Samhain ritual on the day in October when the veil between worlds thins and the dead can reach out and touch you. She's encouraged by her mentor to consider her craft ancestors: mother, grandmother, aunts. Three words come to her during her meditation: "*to—own— myself.*" "I realize," Mar writes, "this is exactly what these women I loved were unable to do themselves: to have own- ership, to each be and own herself completely." Modern Wicca, at its best, is about empowering women. But for an older woman, being called a witch can still stigmatize. "Ditch the witch!" was the chant leveled at the Australian prime minister Julia Eileen Gillard in 2013. And in 2016 anyone with a brain understood that "Lock her up!" was about much more than Hillary Clinton's e-mails.

● ● ●

The exercises in my *Anger Workbook* are remarkably close to witches' spells for releasing anger. The workbook tells me to write out the reasons for my anger on a sheet of paper and then in any way I choose—fire, wind, water—let it go. Both the workbook and the witches' spells I found online encourage me to work out my anger either in a solitary ritual or, better yet, through visualization. In the witches' spells version, after taking a purifying bath and lighting a blue candle, I am instructed to write out the situation that is causing my anger in dove's-blood ink. As the paper catches fire, I am told to chant: "Let peace now enter come and stay, as anger in me goes away."

Another visualization spell instructs me to imagine a ring of white light around my work space as I light a black candle. On a slip of paper, as I conjure a mental picture of the one who has angered me, I am to print their name out in capital letters. Once I burn the paper, in the remaining ash I should write out the emotion I want to replace rage. The *Anger Workbook* goes even further than the casting of the spell. After I visualize myself entering a dark cave, I am told to imagine walking far down inside the earth. There I will meet the person I am furious with. At first I should talk calmly, explaining why I am irate. Afterward I am allowed to imagine screaming, spitting, and punching the person.

◎ ◎ ◎

A surprising number of women felt their first experience of unbridled anger during perimenopause or menopause. One woman felt murderous. "I often felt like I had been body-snatched, and there was a wild ax murderer who took over the control panel of my mind and body." Another felt that it wasn't lessening hormones that made her angry but that menopause lifted the curtain so she could finally see how furious she was. "I distinctly remember looking at a mug of coffee and wanting to throw it against the wall, which was really not something I had ever remotely felt before."

No studies exist that test menopause's connection with anger. Depression, the most common way women experience anger, has been studied. The 2012 SWAN study found a correlation between menopause and depression, while the Melbourne Women's Midlife Health Project, which included not only a survey but also blood tests for estrogen levels, found no direct link. Websites list irritability as a symptom of the change. *Irritability* is a demeaning word, laughably imprecise when what I actually feel is a bright, ascendant rage. I feel indignant that I live in a body, a body that will one day die. "Anger truly felt at its center is the essential living flame of being fully alive and fully here," writes the poet David Whyte. It's an inchoate and electric feeling I recognize from PMS. Menopause and PMS share the same chemical landscape. I was taught not to trust my feelings of frustration and fury in those days before my period when my hormones would drop.

I was told instead that I was crazy, that the world I inhabited was not real.

● ● ●

The supernatural creature women are most often compared to is neither revenant nor witch but the demonically possessed. Partners of menopausal women insist that their wives are not simply going through a hard time but have actually been taken over by a malevolent presence. One husband told a researcher that he wanted the woman he married back—not this awful person she had become. Another said his wife had undergone "a personality transplant." Many call their wives monsters: "She's turned into a crazy monster." "It's like a monster took over her brain." "It's as if an alien had completely taken her over." A man in a chat room wrote that he'd studied up on menopause and even gone to a workshop, but "it did not bring back who she was before."

Angry women are not witches or demonically possessed. They are simply women who are angry. Why is it so hard for the culture to see anger as on a spectrum of female emotions rather than a supernatural infestation? Women too demonize their anger. Online I found several essays written by women that linked their menopausal symptoms to the devil or his minions. In one on *HuffPost* titled "The Difference

Between Menopause and Demonic Oppression," Donna Highfill lists behaviors wrought by "the winged little guys." These include moodiness, lack of self-control, and bursts of anger. "If you're trying to decide," she writes, "if it's menopause or demonic oppression, good luck." Highfill's invocation of demons is tongue-in-cheek, unlike the workshop I found at the website *Finding Freedom. Name* titled "Hormones and Demonic Activity." The deliverance minister Ella LeBain explains the premise of her online class: "What does Adolescence, PMS, Perimenopause and Menopause all have in common? Answer: Hormonal changes attract demonic activity."

This is, of course, insane. I know that demonic possession is a societal construct, not a supernatural reality. Still, I sometimes feel when I wake in the dark, throw off the covers, and wait for the *woomph!* of heat that I am fighting against a force beyond my comprehension and my control. I understand that this force is not speeding toward me like a horror-movie demon from the supernatural sphere but instead resides inside me. I grapple like the women Freud wrote about in his notebooks, women whose bodies became the battleground in society's hysterical repression of the grotesque form.

The grotesque form is both my aging body and my angry self. Dr. Julie Holland got blowback when she suggested in her 2015 book, *Moody Bitches*, that estrogen was the whatever-you-want-honey hormone and that, first during PMS and later in menopause, when the hormonal shroud of accommodation lifts, women should embrace their angry selves. Critics wondered how women, who had to live with and care for others, were supposed to manifest their feelings safely. I get this. It's hard to figure out how to express anger in a world that tells women that anger is unattractive, or as my first husband used to say, unsexy. Furies, the original spirits of anger, had eyes that dripped goo, they threw up clotted blood, and they reeked like a pack of wild dogs. Their anger was "a cancer blasting leaf and child." No wonder even witches' spells encourage women to deal with their anger on their own, better yet using visualization inside their own heads.

Ursula K. Le Guin, the speculative fiction writer, acknowledged that anger was useful in resistance to injustice, but she warned that it's "a tool useful only in combat and self-defense." Le Guin went on to critique the anger used in second-wave feminism: "If feminism was the baby, she's now grown past the stage where her only way to get attention to her needs and wrongs was anger, tantrums, acting out, kicking ass." Only if laws again oppress us do we have the right to access anger. "We're not at that point yet, and I hope nothing we do now brings us closer to it." Dear Ursula: We are at that point. And we have been at that point all along.

"We are living through the moment," the feminist Katha Pollitt wrote in 2017 in *The Nation*, "when women unleash decades of pent-up rage." I've realized with the help of #MeToo and #TimesUp that my anger at my husband and the kitty litter, at the job interviewers who asked who would care for my little daughter if I got the job, and at the harassing boss who continued to be institutionally protected is nearly always rooted in patriarchal oppression. The point of anger is to eventually have less anger. Anger helps me define what I belong to, what I believe in, what I would sacrifice myself for. It helps me deter others from infringing on my rights and focuses my political resistance. If I can work, alongside others, against sexism, my daughter may inherit a world where being female will not hurt quite as much.

"There is a time," Clarissa Pinkola Estés writes in her book *Women Who Run with the Wolves*, "when it becomes imperative to release a rage that shakes the sky. There are times—even though those times are very rare . . . to let loose all the firepower one has."

◉ ◉ ◉

So what happened when I finally got home that rainy night? My husband remembers that he had actually done the dishes and made the bed, a rare occurrence. Mostly he remembers the intensity of my emotions: "I had to hide in my office until you cooled off." I remember the golden quality of the kitchen lamp, how the air itself sparkled with thousands of tiny strobes. I was less a scolding teacher than a lawyer listing off past wrongs. Did he think my job was to clean up after him? Did he suppose that because I was a woman it was my job to deal with cat shit? Was it too much to ask that he close the fucking drawer after he took out a fork, flush the toilet, and not spit in the sink? As I yelled, I felt expansive, as if I were much taller and wider than I actually am. My husband did flee into his office, but to my mind I propelled him through the living room and down the hallway, not with my body but with my mind. I was neither ghost, nor witch, nor medium. I was not a teenage girl in a blood-soaked prom dress. No, I was myself in my mom jeans and teaching sweater, but my rage felt telekinetic as I watched him retreat into his office. I used my will, my own agency, to slam the door.

7 ● The Old Monkey

The *banya* was on rue de la Sourdière in an area of tourist traps selling aprons, tea trays, and coasters printed with the Eiffel Tower. Mike, whose back was sore from the flight over, found the place online. We read that they also offered massages and salt scrubs. A photo beside the services showed red-cheeked men and women smiling at the camera like drunks at an office party. A handwritten note was taped to the *banya* door's wrought-iron filigree that said to call a number to be let inside. A short, plump blonde woman stood beside the door talking on her cell phone in Russian. The woman wore a black strapless dress woven with threads of glittery red, blue, and gold. Her hair was blown out, and though it was hot, she wore a full face of makeup. The woman did not look like someone who'd want a sauna and a massage.

Inside, the hallway was paneled with pine. This was good, reassuring, like the *banya* back home in Brooklyn. We followed the short woman toward the front desk, where unnested Russian dolls were lined up by descending size. A second woman, also blonde but much taller, came out of a back room. It was as if the tall woman were a stretched version of the shorter one. The two had the same yellow hair cut at the shoulders, same doll face, same eyes, removed but at the same time violently cheerful. The tall woman nodded to the short woman, who disappeared into the back room. The tall woman, who wore a short red robe, kissed my husband in the French fashion on each check. When she kissed me, I felt her loose breasts against the bare skin of my clavicle.

If I hadn't been so disoriented, the feel of the tall woman's body might have given me a sexual jolt. But beyond my current confusion, sex, which had held me under its spell for thirty years, was now slowly receding. Its signal, once distinct, was now so soft it was hardly audible at all.

The tall woman moved behind the desk and pulled out a xeroxed piece of paper in a plastic sleeve. Under a photo of a woman, it read 50 euros including a steam. Under a photo of a man, it said 120 euros. I asked why it was so much more for a man. The tall woman looked at me and then at my husband. I could tell her first impression of us had disintegrated into something else. "Because," she said, "it is for man."

Inside the dark sauna we spread our towels on the hot wood. We'd put on our bathing suits, to the obvious amusement of the tall woman. "What is this place?" I asked. Mike laughed and said, "I have no idea." So many years of police reporting had numbed his sense of the absurd. He lifted a pale arm into the air, then bent it behind his back, stretching. He was enjoying the heat. I said, "Do you think it's a massage parlor?" He switched arms, his glasses totally fogged up. "Maybe," he said. "Do you want to leave?" I did. But I also felt embarrassed. Here we were, two nitwit American tourists. Also I couldn't quite believe it was a massage parlor. I'd fantasized about such places, and to find myself not in imagination but physically inside one felt both unreal and portentous. The door swung open then and a naked man entered. Around his middle hung a thick doughnut of flesh. Below, like coconuts held in nylon, his heavy genitalia. He settled himself in the corner and stared at Mike and me as if he'd never seen humans before.

In a Parisian sauna just like this one, the art critic Catherine Millet, author of *The Sexual Life of Catherine M*, writes about taking many men at once: "I had alternately bent and reached up to take all the eager pricks in my mouth." That scene of orgy now superimposed itself over this moment of awkwardness. What, if anything, was supposed to happen? I was getting hot, and not just from the air that emanated from the metal contraption in the corner where electrical embers glowed. I was moving into the aura before a flash. Normal reality floated away through space like the lost panel on a starship; then the heat rose like fire rolling along a wire. Mike emphatically had not wanted a massage, while I'd felt pressured into getting a massage as well as a sauna. Now I just wanted this all to be over.

I stood, said I was going to have my massage, slipped out of the heat, and walked down the hall to the front desk, where the tall blonde woman was reading a paperback and listening to techno music. The short woman had changed into the *banya*'s signature red mini-robe and was sitting on the floor against the wall, still talking on her cell phone. Her toenails were painted neon orange. I said I was ready for my massage. The tall woman looked at me as if she'd forgotten the money that had changed hands. But then she smiled deeply, her lips cutting up into her cheeks. She said something sharp in Russian. The short woman jumped up and walked quickly down the hallway. She pulled off her robe, hung it on a hook. Her body, while not thin, was young and lovely. Her breasts swayed a little but her nipples were large, puffy, and between her legs there was no hair at all, just a slit of deep, grainy pink. I watched her yank the sauna door open and disappear inside.

● ● ●

Her body reminded me of the first body, besides those of my family, I'd seen. After a movie at the Cineplex and a

Pizza Hut pizza, my high school boyfriend and I lay on a plaid blanket under a yellow school bus parked in a Baptist church lot. After making out for an hour, a bobbing pink object emerged just below his waist. The cock seemed unconnected to his body, crude, unfinished, like a lump of elongated clay.

You might think that coming of age in the 1970s, as I did, the perks of the sexual revolution would have trickled down into my physical life. You would be wrong. Free love was on television, something far away and consistently denigrated by my mother. I remember fixating on John Denver, Bobby Sherman, my best friend Mandy Messner's feet encased in lacy white ankle socks. Also hard rain, lying in a patch of moss, bubble baths. I'd heard of masturbation, but only as something that boys did. I don't think I knew women could self-stimulate, make themselves come. Sexy was on the outside, not on the inside. Sex was something a man started up with you; it wasn't an intrinsic inner reality. I thought of my vagina, when I thought of it at all, as a blankness, a void. I was like my childhood doll—if ripped open, there'd be nothing, a hollow, an empty space.

My sexuality developed in the hothouse of my mother's negativity. Like a lot of women in the '50s, before the pill made premarital sex less dangerous, she'd been taught that sex outside marriage could ruin a woman, that desire should be pressed down, that only slutty girls enjoyed sex. Free love confused and frightened her. In our one and only sex talk, she told me that intercourse was disgusting, that the sperm ran down your legs. When I was late for my curfew or wore a top that showed too much cleavage or midriff, or shorts that did not cover enough thigh, my mother, confronted with my teen-age sexuality, lost it.

Her negativity did not keep me from having sex, but it did, for a long time, keep me from enjoying it. After I lost my virginity, I locked myself in the bathroom of the apartment my college boyfriend shared with two other friends. I had lied to my parents, said I was sleeping over at a girlfriend's house, and driven two hours on the highway to be with him. This level of duplicity was new for me. I was light-headed. I cried as I hugged the toilet while throwing up my dinner and eventually yellow bile. I remember how the shower curtain hung by only a few hooks and had a lattice of black, lacelike mold along its hem. What had I done? I'd cut myself off from my mother and my family, violently and forever, and entered the stream of a greater force that I knew I could never control. I was aware of sex's overwhelming power. Its disorienting chaos: "What a human being possesses deep within him," Georges Bataille writes, "of the loss of the tragic, of the blinding world, can be found again nowhere but in bed." My boyfriend tried to get me to come out, but I fell asleep on the floor. I woke to muzzy light coming from the frosted-glass window and the sound of my boyfriend again saying my name from behind the locked door.

I am not focusing here on men or my relationship to them but on the history of this body, my legs, my arms, my mouth, my cunt. What it wanted, how afraid it was, how it moved relentlessly forward, how it was sometimes cowardly, other times brave.

It wasn't until the summer after college, when I finally touched myself and began to fantasize outside the physical reality of intercourse, that my sexual life improved. My first time masturbating was the opposite of the horror of the first cock I'd seen under the bus or the anxiety of losing my virginity. House-sitting in Washington, D.C., I was flipping around on the channels when I landed on a woman in a transparent dress, her hands pressed between her legs. Behind her was a swirl of moving color, like the hallucinatory montages in '60s movies. Blood flowed into my lower body and I tightened, as I did when making out. I put my own hand between my legs. Within a few strokes I came, going off convulsively, like a windup toy.

In relation with myself I learned the nuances of my body and grew conversant with my inner sexual landscape. Sex became less stressed. Oddly, by not being completely present, I could be so much more passionate and engaged. When I met the man who was to be my first husband, we had sex every single night. I remember how the pressure built between my legs during the day, and how in the evening my future husband

and I fucked on the terrible mattress of a fold-out couch. Sex was the force that bracketed my days, kept my life's narrative in order. Rising desire, fulfilled desire, over and over, day after day.

The hours spent on that fold-out couch have a warmth and completeness unlike any of my other sexual memories. It's an irony to me that during the hours I was the most sexually worked up, literally dizzy with desire, I was also the coziest and felt the safest. I was sated, warm, expansive. Unsure where my body ended and my future husband's began. Romantic bonding uses the same pathways and chemicals as mother-child bonding. Oxytocin drives both systems, and the neurological programs are identical. During those long Saturday afternoons when I got out of bed only to pee or heat up a little soup, I was brought back to my earliest sensation of pleasure: the drugged exquisiteness of pressing up against my mother's warm skin.

◎ ◎ ◎

Back in Paris, the tall woman in the red robe told me to call her Katrina and pulled back the velvet curtain. I stepped into a cellar room with a vaulted ceiling, a room you might envision as a monk's cell described in a Gothic novel. Dimly lit, damp, it had in the far corner a table that held what I first thought was a whip but then realized was a black extension cord. To get here, I'd followed Katrina down a narrow spiral stairwell into a long, dark hallway that smelled strongly of sperm. The smell brought back the old man I'd seen the one and only time I'd gone to a New York City sex club. All night I'd watched him under the black light, wandering around like a lost child in a diaper and a pair of bunny slippers.

Over the mantel was a large black-and-white poster of a naked woman. She was thin, her eyes vacant behind a feather mask. The poster board the image was mounted on had bowed a little and had what I hoped was a water stain in one corner. It wasn't until I saw the photo that I finally accepted that I was in a place where women took money for sex.

Katrina told me to take off my bathing suit and lie facedown on the table, and she left the room. I heard her walking away down the hallway, her steps getting faint. I pulled my suit off, crawled up on the massage table, and lay facedown, head in the table's hole. I tried to arrange a towel that did not seem completely clean over my bare ass. What the fuck had I gotten myself into? On the table, I felt completely without erotic energy. Maybe it was anxiety or embarrassment, but I felt my sexuality was buried or lost.

Early times of sexual frenzy seem almost impossible now. After my first marriage ended when I was in my late thirties, I had a few months of frenetic sex. I'd burned down my life and, like a crazed survivor, I'd bashed my way into one bed after another, each encounter both acute and fleeting: a man kneeling behind me, rooted inside; a friend-turned-lover asking to come on my face. These encounters, while erotic, were also unconnected and ephemeral, like beads flown off a broken chain. In throwing myself at bodies, I was trying to trigger forth new life, but using this method I was unable to make anything new happen.

During that time, as my first marriage ended, I fantasized violently. The sexual act took on an almost mechanical intensity. Cocks pistoled into pink holes. Words that during the daylight hours would hurt me I loved hearing in the dark.

"Your hole OK?" *My hole?* "Your head not hurt?" Katrina meant the hole in the massage table my face was jammed into. Fine, I said. I tried to sound businesslike and keep very still. I wanted to make clear to her that I was here for a regular massage, the kind a ginger man with a bird tattoo gave me back in Brooklyn. Katrina started a two-finger poke down my spine, like a novice playing "Chopsticks" on the piano. It was clear she had no idea how to give an unsexy massage. Even now I don't understand why I didn't get up politely and say that my stomach hurt or that I had a sudden headache. I didn't want to hurt Katrina's feelings. She was obviously uncomfortable as she tried in her rudimentary English to be kind, asking about stress and how much I slept each night. I wasn't sure if she thought I was a debauched housewife, wanting group sex in the sauna, or a resigned wife accepting of her sex-crazed husband's dirty fantasies. Maybe she'd figured out we'd misunderstood the website and so, to keep cover, was pretending everything was normal. I began to worry about what the short blonde-haired woman was doing to my husband inside the sauna.

I tried to remember the last time Mike and I had had sex. It had been at least a month and maybe more. Before I met him, in the sad wake after my first marriage ended, I'd regularly prayed: *Send me someone good to love. I promise not to fuck it up this time.*

Since early adulthood, desire had been the main way I'd oriented myself. Without it, I often feel now that I've lost the thread. When I go to a party, I no longer rank the men in order of fuckability. I don't feel desire accumulate day after day until my pussy is buzzed, jittery. It's not that my husband isn't attractive. He is. His pale blue eyes are set off by salt-and-pepper hair, and he has very nice legs. He's self-deprecating and funny. But it was as if between me and my longing, a thick pane of frosted glass had been erected.

Lying on the table, I felt Katrina, using one finger, jab at my shoulder. I wondered if my husband had known this was a brothel all along. Maybe he'd planned to come here and have sex with someone other than me. We sometimes told our fantasies to each other, and he'd had a few that had taken place in an erotic space like this one. I regretted how closed I'd been to him lately. When I flashed, he brought me ice packs from the refrigerator, and he put up with our bedroom's cold temperature—both in winter, when I'd leave the window open, and in summer, when I'd blast the air-conditioning. I'd acted like my body was a room I didn't want to get messed up. I'd shut myself off. During our trip to Paris I felt a sensation of coming up short, a sort of running out, like pulling the last piece of tape off a roll and being left with no way to bind things together.

"Tumble over," Katrina said. Tumble down was more like it. I was in free fall, like Alice down her hole, falling past not clocks and doors but dildos and handcuffs. Imagining my husband with the short woman I'd seen go into the sauna, just a girl, really, her lovely breasts and the pink of her skin warmed by the sauna. I moved the two of them around in my head like Barbie and Ken dolls in one position after another. Worst, when I went in for a close-up, was the expression of gratitude on my husband's face.

◎ ◎ ◎

In menopause I often find myself ejected from my own fantasies. Not a central and desired player but a bystander at best jealous and at worst dejected and betrayed. Several of the menopausal women I spoke with told me they had traded fantasies of their own degradation for ones of their partners with younger women. "I used to have rape fantasies, but now they have been replaced with walking into a room and seeing my husband sitting on a couch with a college-age girl straddling him," one woman said. "She's always skinny with small, firm breasts and dark hair. He has one hand on the back of her head and the other fingering her anus."

In the psychoanalytical study *Change of Life*, the therapist Ann Mankowitz follows her patient Rachel through menopause. Rachel dreams about a burnt-out house. Her loss of fertility feels sudden: "First there was the shock to her mind; she felt as though she had woken up from a deep sleep to find that part of her was dead." Midway through her treatment Rachel admits to fantasies that Markowitz calls masochistic. "They were truly so that the pain of them enhanced her own sexual pleasure." Rachel sees her husband as a lecherous old man and herself as a young girl. "Sometimes she matched him in lechery, sometimes she was resistant—while the part of herself that was the middle-aged matriarch watched, excited by jealousy." The fantasies that disturb Rachel the most are the ones where she is left out completely, "excluded from the erotic dyad."

It seems perverse to feed off an image of my own betrayal. Maybe so. But clearly I'm not the only woman who has erotized what hurt her. In their book *Private Thoughts*, the sex therapist Wendy Maltz and the journalist Suzie Boss found that many of the women they interviewed had sexualized traumatic experiences. One woman, when she drew a blue-print of her violent fantasy, realized it was the bedroom where her grandfather had molested her. Another woman's fantasies are fixated on an older man having sex with a young girl; while the characters vary, the scenario replicates her own early abuse by an uncle.

These women erotize an early trauma, I an imaginary one. Scientists believe that our ability to spontaneously lubricate at the sight of almost anything even slightly sexual was selected to protect us from tearing and infection. I'd argue that fantasy serves a similar, though emotional, function as a sort of coping mechanism, a way to incorporate, deactivate, and erotize what we find most frightening.

Celia, nearing fifty, worried about the appeal of her aging body. She told me that she often obsessed over women younger than herself. A young male friend confided to Celia that his wife's vagina was too tight, that it was hard for them to have intercourse. In the weeks that followed, Celia found herself fixating on men fucking young women with tight vaginas. Tightness became a sensation she relished, but one that, after giving birth to her two children, she did not possess. She felt the fantasy lacked self-esteem. Celia tried to stop, but the image was like a magnet pulling her back. She even googled "how to get rid of an unwanted fantasy" but found little help. The solution finally came from an unexpected source: gay porn. "It was all cock," she told me, "and no pussy." For Celia, the porn worked like a reset button. Watching men have sex was a palate-cleansing sorbet that wiped out her fixation on men and their tight-pussied partners and let her place her own body back in the center of her fantasy life.

◎ ◎ ◎

There is the mind and, nestled like an egg in its nest, the erotic imagination, but there is also the body. During menopause the vagina comes under medical and sexual surveillance. Not since virginity has there been so much interest in its fleshy realities. Like the breasts, the cunt is an organ that, while a part of my body, is also judged communally. I remember my mother, her voice shaky with outrage, telling me that she'd heard a man on television, a man in line to get into a strip club, say, "I don't know what the big deal is? It looks like an oyster and it smells like one too." His remark aimed at devaluing what had so much power over him. Vaginas are both physical and metaphorical. Unsettled places. Liminal openings that exist not in a brick railway station wall or the back of a wardrobe but in our own bodies.

I thought the origin of the word *vagina* might hint at its mutability, its position as conduit to all new life. I was wrong. The word *vagina* comes from the Latin *vagina*, which means "sheath for a sword." I've often felt oppressed by the sheer multitude of pliable pornographic pussies. Their openness.

Their velvet complicity. These are the qualities, from a cultural standpoint, that define the ideal cunt. Women, though, have often wished for an organ with more intrinsic agency. In William Faulkner's *Sanctuary*, Temple Drake fantasizes that her own genitalia might become aggressive: "I was thinking maybe it would have long sharp spikes on it and he wouldn't know until it was too late."

As a girl, I found solace in the image of the vagina dentata, the toothed vagina. From my first awareness of the hole between my legs, the pink lips, I'd wondered if, like my mouth, my vagina might one day speak. Tales of the vagina dentata mostly read as male castration fears. There is the Maori myth in which the trickster Mauri turns himself into a penis-like worm. As he tries to wriggle inside the Night Goddess Hine-nui-te-po, she awakens and bites him with her obsidian vaginal teeth. In another account, written by a priest during the time of the Inquisition, a witch keeps the penises her vagina has severed in a wooden box. Inside the box the penises move around loudly, waiting to be fed their daily dose of corn.

A toothed vagina, by reason, is attached to a castrating bitch. But as Tina Fey has said, bitches get shit done. At the Brooklyn Museum, less than a mile from my house, Judy Chicago's *The Dinner Party* imagines the vaginas of thirty-nine historically important women, from Susan B. Anthony, the queen of the table, whose ovoid hole is fenestral black, to Virginia

Woolf, whose meat-petal labia rise up around the stones she put into her pockets to drown herself.

Chicago's vaginas, like horror-movie villains, look a bit unhinged. Violently generative, some even have cowry-shell teeth. Teeth or not hardly matter, though, because these depictions have nothing to do with pornographic fuckability. Hilton Kramer, the late art critic, called *The Dinner Party* "failed bad art" in "abysmal taste." I bet he'd never, as I have, sat in a birthing class where a would-be father asked if after pregnancy his wife's vagina would go back to its original tightness. I do wish, though, that he could have heard the birth instructor's Chicago-like reply. "No," she said, "but by then hopefully you'll be mature enough to handle it."

◎ ◎ ◎

Vaginas are not static. They are malleable, elastic; during birth they blow up to several times their normal size. Once fertility is over, the vagina transitions again. The walls may thin; lubrication can lessen. While age can affect the materiality of the vagina, it has no direct effect on the biology of arousal. Desire still releases dopamine, capillaries in the genitals still swell with blood, and the area of the brain just behind the left eye that is linked with reason and control still shuts down. Blood and electricity shoot into the cerebellum and the frontal cortex. Cells discharge oxytocin, which leads to pelvic-floor contractions, followed by uterine and vaginal contractions. It's never been conclusively proven that decreased hormones affect desire in any way. Yet according to medical studies, nearly half of all women complain of low desire as they move through menopause. Hypoactive sexual desire dysfunction (HSDD) is the medical term for female low desire. Factors that make women vulnerable are depression and exhaustion. The most predictable similarity among women who have HSDD, though, is that they are partnered.

Around fifty, when entered, I felt a fullness, a tightness I remembered from my first few sexual acts as a teenager. Even with lube, intercourse was not comfortable; it was as if I'd traveled back through time to the very beginning of my sex life, before intercourse was normalized, when it was still a little painful and very strange.

Orgasms, while no more elusive, have in sensation also changed. The clitoris spreads down from the little nub, known as the glans, into a large mass of sensitive tissue, the root. From there, bulbs attached to dozens of thread-thin legs stretch out inside the body. The clit is a star configuration fanning like a fish skeleton around the uterus. In menopause climaxes vary in both velocity and gradation. Some stars surge, others flicker, and a few are completely blown out.

The most common complaint in menopausal chat rooms is that penetration hurts. "I have low libido and vaginal dryness, so sex is not fun at all," one woman said. Another woman noted a burning sensation: "I felt like my vagina was ripping open as if giving birth." One old friend told me sex hurts and that she now understands the term "wifely duty." Another told me that she could not imagine enjoying a penis being thrust into her. "If old people are doing it," she said, "I'd like to know how." A gynecologist I interviewed told me that her patients don't care if intercourse is enjoyable; they just don't want it to be painful. They want to "give" their husbands spontaneous moisture and pliability, even if they have to be medicated to do so.

The psychologist Lisa M. Diamond writes in her 2014 book *Sexual Fluidity* that pharmaceutical companies are feverishly searching for a treatment for HSDD, "yet the more we learn about women's desires, the more obvious it becomes that they involve complex interplays among biological, environmental, psychological, and interpersonal factors." Diamond reports that "relationship context appears to be particularly important to women, so much so that some clinicians have suggested reframing the term 'low sexual desire' as 'a desire discrepancy' between partners. After all," she writes, "maybe a woman's sex drive seems low only when her partner wants sex more often than she does. If that is the case, who has the problem?"

Women too, at least heterosexual ones, privilege intercourse. I know this because for much of my life, fucking was the center of my sexual universe. For me, the drama of sex moved in frenetic rushes of desire toward penetration. I liked oral sex, but I thought of it as prelude only, not the main course. To have a cock rooted inside me, to feel the pulse, the warm spurt, and to go off just after. I thought of coming together as a hook, as if the proximity of orgasm made an actual material link that bound me to my partner. I won't deny that the pleasure was intense, euphoric. But I also know I privileged intercourse in part because the culture in general did. I wanted to be fuckable. Also I was drawn to moody, uncommunicative men who could be best reached through intercourse, and the surest way to make that connection was through the cultural ideal of simultaneous orgasm.

Enter my second husband, Mike, he of the thin hips and odd hairy wrist mole. Our first night together we moved along the familiar sexual script toward intercourse, but once our bodies connected, I felt not rising excitement in him but a lull. It wasn't that the act bored him; it was more an excited but neutral phase. I kept trying with my hips, the pressure of my weight, my mouth, to get him to ignite, to focus our energy together toward the summit. But he pulled out and we moved on to other positions. At first I was confused. Was there something wrong with me? Was there something wrong with him? After a month I asked him if he didn't like intercourse. He looked startled. "I love it," he said, "but I love other things just as much."

For a long time I felt frustrated and even a little bitter about this. A few times early in our relationship he accused me of checking out during sex. He was right. Without fucking being central, I felt let down, and in passive-aggressive protest, I would zone out. As time passed, though, I realized my pleasure was no less than in my early phallic-centered sexual life and actually greater. As more time passed and I entered menopause, with its sexual changes, I realized how lucky I was that intercourse had been uprooted from its central position.

◉ ◉ ◉

Some women prop up intercourse with lube or hormonal treatments. Others open up what it means to be physical. A small but enthusiastic group stops having sex altogether. For those women, celibacy brings freedom. One said, "A lot of men my age have spent their lives being in charge—and I don't want anyone behaving as if they are in charge of me. Loss of libido is a really small price to pay for autonomy." Another woman told me that while she masturbates occasionally, she never thinks about sex. "At first in my forties I was afraid not to think about it, thought I was losing something important. Now I just feel relieved."

Susan, a fifty-five-year-old artist and mother of two, told me the movement away from sex was gradual: "It happened slowly without either my husband or I initiating the (̶ sation. It was natural." Susan felt that sex was bec̲ ̲ ̲ ̲ ̲ stressful. "It felt compulsory, routine-like. Also when I was not in the mood, it was painful." Now she feels unburdened. "It's so much better, as I don't have to feel guilt or give an excuse, because it is not expected." Susan feels her connection with her husband is much deeper than physicality. "Not having sex doesn't in any way reduce the way we feel about each other. There was a time for it, and maybe now it is time to do other things."

Celibacy, in a sex-crazed culture, is the most debased form of sexuality. And while celibacy has had ruinous effects when it is enforced institutionally, after a long sexual life a percentage of women, small but content, see it as a way to get out of the sexual rat race. In her book *A History of Celibacy*, Elizabeth Abbott writes that celibacy is a way to love many people at once without being unfaithful to any of them. Abbott points at celibacy's long ties to spirituality, how at Delphi, the Pythia, or female priest, had to be at least fifty and completely celibate: "Apollo could not enter a body blocked by sexual pleasure." Finally, though, it's not divinity but peace that celibacy engenders. "Our eroticism is not tied solely to heterosexual intercourse or reproduction," Abbott writes. "We can reclaim our sexuality without turning the world upside down; we can, through celibacy and masturbation, define our own sexuality and satisfy ourselves."

Celibacy, for most of the women I talked to, was out of the question either because of their own desire or their partner's, or both. While some do not enjoy the act and feel forced to comply, more have expanded their idea of what it means to be sexual. "I have gained the wisdom as I aged," one woman told me, "that all our bodies are different, that the media has distorted what a real body looks like, and that most men are just thrilled to have a naked woman in their bed." Another woman taught her partner to use a vibrator, which she calls "life-changing." Many discover a late-life interest in sex acts other than intercourse. One single woman, a stylist, felt that menopause ramped up her sexuality. She discovered anal sex and began to date younger, less uptight men. Through them she realized she was still attractive. "Maybe not in the same way I was in my twenties and thirties, but that's all right," she said. "There are several seasons to a woman's sexual attractiveness. No need to look like you're twenty or get Botox. Sexuality is way deeper than superficial looks."

Even my most sexually adventurous friend, fifty-two-year-old Mercedes, a San Francisco fabric designer, has slowed down a little: "I don't have those afternoons anymore when my body is screaming for sex." When her daughter was young, Mercedes felt she had to censor herself, but now that her daughter is at college, Mercedes is "putting herself back together again." Mercedes still goes to sex parties, but instead of pursuing the acts she once savored—S&M, swapping, sleeping with much younger men—she is now more interested in voyeurism: "Now I get turned on by watching." Still, whether it's with a partner or by masturbating, she likes to come at least once a day to "detox" but also for the chance to get out from under her own consciousness. "In orgasm I'm like a ringing bell," she tells me. "And afterwards for an hour or so, I'm not quite me—I feel outside myself."

Of the half dozen men I spoke to who had menopausal partners, many were frustrated by their wives' changing attitude toward sex. They deflected questions about their own aging bodies and were focused instead on their wives' libido. One man told me his wife no longer wanted to have sex with him; she had told him to go elsewhere. "This breaks a bond," he said. Another man said that while his day-to-day relationship with his wife was steadier, he did miss their old sex life: "I do sometimes long for how it was before, no doubt about it." Another man, a professor in his sixties, told me that his wife's sex drive had diminished: "Now we have less sex but more hugging, hand-holding, and kissing." Another man, a freelance writer in his late fifties, found more positive than negative in postmenopausal sex. Sex, he told me, is now more like play. "That doesn't mean that there can't be or isn't intensity and urgency—just that sex doesn't seem as apocalyptic as it once might have been." The underlying knowledge that a child could come from sex was weighty. Birth control did not do away with that subterranean sense. After menopause there is a relinquishing of stakes. "It takes us back to play and a different, more luxurious relationship with time."

One woman I spoke to, a sixty-four-year-old lesbian who works in film production, said she too feels a postmenopausal sexual freedom. "One of the best things about being a lesbian," she told me, "is that I was able to be myself and still find romantic love. This is more true now than ever." She does have a weaker libido, but because her wife is also in her early sixties, this is not a problem. "We would never put sexual pressure on one another." Jane and PJ, a lesbian couple in their early fifties, are more melancholy about the changes that menopause brings. Their sex life has mellowed. "We don't have the same range," PJ said. "We're not, like, strapping dildos on and fucking each other against the refrigerator." While sex is less frequent and intense, it is now more satisfying. The couple have been together a long time, and they know each other's bodies completely. "We have sex less," Jane said, "but we enjoy it more."

◉ ◉ ◉

I'd argue that it's the call to authenticity that menopause provokes, the urge to root out segments of life that are fraudulent, that at least in part upset and realign sexual life. "The aging woman," Simone de Beauvoir writes, "well knows that if she ceases to be an erotic object, it is not only because her flesh no longer has fresh bounties for men; it is also because her past, her experience, make her, willy-nilly, a person; she has struggled, loved, willed, suffered, enjoyed, on her own account. This independence is intimidating."

◎ ◎ ◎

I can embrace my body's transition, realize there is nothing tragic in using a little lube, feel that an earlier fragmentation created by cycling and the male gaze is finally mending. I can sense, as I sometimes do, that I am back where I was before menstruation—a fierce girl ready to take on the world. The thing I can't change is the sexual disgust the greater culture aims at older women. Sooner or later I will become a body not only invisible but also despised.

There is no manifestation of sexual repulsion for female flesh more visceral than the bathroom scene in *The Shining*. Jack Nicholson is drawn to room 237 in the Overlook Hotel. The bathroom there is green, fecund, leaf-like. The shower curtain shifts, and a young woman steps out of the tub. Nicholson's face, as he watches, moves from trepidation into his signature expression; chin lowered, eyes aslant, a smile as malevolent as it is lustful. As they kiss, worry creeps into Jack's features. When he opens his eyes, he sees in the mirror the woman's back, not young and smooth but wrinkled, sagging, with patches of soft, brown-colored flesh. Jack springs back and runs from the bathroom, through the bedroom, and out the front door.

I had to watch this footage ten times before I became desensitized to the disgust that blocks out the old woman's power. Smiling, arms reaching out, she understands that Jack is unable to see her, or any woman, as anything but a sex object and that her sudden emergence has thrown him into wild, chaotic repulsion. She knows his horror is not of her age but of the material law itself. Forced to create the illusion that growth stops in the first decade or two of adult female life, the old woman is nearly giddy now that the mask is off and she is finally free. Interwoven with the chase are scenes of the old woman rising up out of the bathtub. Her hair is short and she looks, while rotting, oddly elegant. We understand what Jack can't: that the crone doesn't replace the young woman, that all our previous ages stay tucked inside us. We are old women, young mothers, and small girls. The young woman is essentially the same as the old one, the seed buried inside a wrinkled fruit.

◉ ◉ ◉

Is it our aging female bodies that disgust or the familiarity engendered by our long-term relationships? The Kinsey Reports posit that humans are not the only species that becomes "psychologically fatigued" with long-term partners. "Among monkeys it has been noted that animals caged together gradually become less aroused by each other, preliminary sex play must be extended before they are stimulated enough to attempt coitus, and the subsequent copulation is less vigorous." Of course when a new monkey, no matter its age, enters the cage, all the old monkeys want to have sex with him or her. "Foreplay time shortens and copulation is vigorous."

Everybody wants to fuck the new monkey. The new monkey, unlike the old monkey, is not yet aware that you leave your used dental floss all over the floor, that you regularly and repeatedly stain the couch with pen ink. They don't yet know the depression you feel after you speak to your mother on the phone or how chronic hives have you scratching your feet all night. Fucking the new monkey has that lack of context that is often called sexy.

Jonathan Huber, an MD and a researcher in Canada, told me that unlearning is the most important part of remaining sexually vital in later life. Unlearning is key to loving both the old monkey that is our partner and the old monkey that is our self. In an ongoing long-term study of older couples who continue to have what Huber calls "great sex," participants told him that the way to sexual vibrancy was to welcome our own and our partner's authentic self. What might someone unlearn in order to move toward authenticity? "Basically everything society and culture tells you about sex," Huber told me. "Much of the information we pick up along the way is contradictory, negative, or just downright incorrect. Examples might be people who have a lot of sex are bad, women should orgasm as a result of vaginal penetration, masturbation is dirty and shameful, the only good sex is spontaneous, sex has to result in orgasm for both parties at the same time."

● ● ●

Great sex was the last thing on my mind in Paris as Katrina told me the massage was over and left me alone to get dressed. I sat up dazed, not with relaxation but with extreme anxiety. I felt as if I'd stumbled into the shabby back room of my own fantasy and was finally able to see an early sexual self, a woman who had fetishized the gender binary as well as more conventional aspects of the erotic life. Like O, in *The Story of O*, I'd often gotten off on self-negation, wanting to be a zero, an emptiness, in an almost religious attempt to transcend myself. As soon as I got an honest look at my earlier self, she was gone, receding like a loosed balloon, higher and higher into the heavens. I felt a little sad to see her go. While she'd had some messed-up ideas, she'd also, in her thigh-highs and push-up bra, given me a lot of pleasure.

As I pulled my bathing suit back on, I felt tender, wobbly-legged, vulnerable. The circular stairwell was like a corkscrew birth canal. At the front desk there was no sign of Katrina. I walked past the metal lockers where we'd stored our clothes and shoes, then around the corner to the sauna. There was so much blood pulsating in my ears I felt woozy. Would I find inside the sauna a scenario that would prove my body had been replaced by a younger, more pliable one? I pulled the door open, the heat hit me like I'd opened an oven door, and it took my eyes a moment to adjust to the dimmer light. There was no sign of the short blonde woman, who, my husband told me later, had left cheerfully after both he and the fat man had said they did not want a massage.

Mike was pink and glittery with sweat. He radiated an animal immanence that was, frankly, intoxicating. I felt an unbearable longing for my old monkey, his chaotic chest hair, his giant big toes, the swell of his belly. I wanted Mike less as a man than as a human. I wanted the disembodied part of Mike, the one I am getting to know as we age. He was relieved to see me too, reaching out for my hand, pulling me down beside him, and throwing a sweaty arm around my waist. He introduced the fat man as Marcel. Marcel was a botanist who studied ferns. "I was just telling him," Mike said in his gentle Southern drawl, "how beautiful the Blue Ridge Mountains are in spring."

8 ● Nocturnal Hunter

In the last raw days of winter I find myself wide awake in the dark, trying not to disturb my husband sleeping beside me. I shift, freeze in one position after another. Finally I go downstairs, turn on the kitchen faucet, and get a glass of water. Looking out the back window into the yard, I see that the bare branches of the oak tree are like ink drops rolled every which way on paper. In an upper window of the house across the way, blue flows like a lava lamp behind a curtain. I open the hall closet and get out the box of my mother's papers. I've had the box since I closed down her house five years ago, but only lately have I heard, like a faint heartbeat, the box signaling to me.

In the dark, I think of my mother in the years our relationship was at its worst. I was a teenager and she was in her late forties when she stalked our un-air-conditioned Virginia ranch house wearing only a slip, her face red and covered in sweat. When I asked what was wrong, she'd say nothing. I often found her sitting on the stairs in the only cool place, the unfinished basement, sobbing so hard she could hardly catch her breath.

I've always wanted my mother in the dark. When I cried out from my crib, my mother said, I settled down if she brought me into her bed. As a child, when I would go into my parents' dark room and get in bed on my mother's side, I wanted to feel her skin, her warmth, her vast oceanic presence enveloping me. I wanted to feel, as I must have longed to do as an infant, that we were one.

Inside the box, I find an envelope of pictures of my parents' wedding. Their second wedding—the first was a quick courtroom affair held six weeks earlier, just after my mother found out she was pregnant. At the reception after the second wedding, my father is blond and boyish in his clericals. His black minister suit coat hangs on his thin frame. My mother wears a knee-length white satin dress, gloves, and pearls. Her veil falls in folds of netting around her face. She is twenty years old, flushed and beautiful. The pictures are like a million others from the early 1960s. They cut the cake, feed slices to each other. What fascinates me is not my parents' youth but what is not there, or more precisely, what's not yet visible. Inside my mother's body, in the space above and between her legs, a tiny creature no bigger than a pinkie fingernail. A clump of cells on a mission. Me.

On our last evening together, I made my mother a roast chicken with vegetables, which I served on a bare table. The thrift-store plates, the mismatched silver, the paper napkins, the terrible blankness of the white enamel tabletop. The rawness of the table continues to haunt me. For our last meal, couldn't I have used my good plates and put a cloth on the table? After dinner she wanted to watch the television show *Downton Abbey*, about a lord and his family in the early 1900s. She'd always loved everything about rich people. To my mother, money, which she never had much of, was an object of adoration. This adoration was not tainted by greed but was pure, almost religious in nature. I didn't have a TV, only my laptop. I suggested we watch the Will Ferrell movie *Elf*. She sneered—a movie about a grown man pretending to be a Christmas elf?

Midway through the movie, she took a photo out of her wallet. It was an image of my wedding to Mike the spring before. I stood smiling under the Oriental Pavilion in Prospect Park in my pink silk wedding dress. The photo was taken just after the ceremony, and though it was a gray day, I am clearly euphoric. "Do you notice anything?" my mother asked, her voice moving toward a familiar self-righteousness. I looked again. I knew my happiness was not what she wanted me to see. She had always spoken out against elaborate second weddings, saying they were inappropriate, tacky. I'd always assumed she was jealous, as she herself had not had a second marriage. She was also angry that men tended to remarry much younger women. But Mike and I were the same age. Our wedding modest. I looked again at my silver cage sandals, pale legs, the pink silk dress, my hair up in a loose bun. Did my mother think the dress was too young for me? At forty-nine, I was a menopausal bride. "Your pubic hair is showing," my mother finally said.

At first I thought I'd misheard her. I looked at the photo. Under the dress, I'd worn a thick beige bodysuit and control-top tights. I knew for a fact that there was no way my pubic hair could be showing. "It's just a shadow in the material," I said. My mother shook her head and said, "I don't think so." She stuck the photo inside the slit of her purse. I felt light-headed, numb, furious. She continued to complain about the loss of *Downton Abbey* until *Elf* was over and we both went to bed.

I've come out of my mother's body three times. Once when I was born; once in adolescence, a baby woman breaking out of the maternal crust; and when she died, I came out a final time. The times before this last time, though I was outside, I was also partly inside her. But now that she's dead, I've come out completely. This is why, just after she died, I felt so exposed. As if for the first time I was abandoned under the huge dome of sky. Unprotected. Now that I'm finally out, I'm trying to see her and also to consume her. I can't be inside her anymore. Now I must work to get her inside me.

In Toni Morrison's novel *Jazz*, self-ownership is what heals fifty-year-old Violet's fragmented self, an ownership reached only by finally having compassion for her own menopausal mother: "Mama, Mama? Is this where you got to and couldn't do it no more? The place of shade without trees where you know you are not and never again will be loved by anybody who can choose to do it?"

"What does one discover," Elena Ferrante was asked, "in freeing the body of the mother from shapelessness?" Frankly I have no idea. It's been five years since my mother died, and then, many days later, the police found her body naked on the living room floor. In the years since her death I've contemplated her monstrousness, her witch-like power. I'd dismissed her pain as outsize bitterness. But that is too easy, reductive. I see that my mother and I must go another round. Otherwise she won't stay buried. Already her fingertips are reaching up out of the dirt, trying to grab on to my own.

Lessened progesterone may be responsible for menopausal insomnia, though this, like most menopause speculation, has yet to be proven conclusively. Some studies show that it's hot flashes that wake women in the night and keep them awake. Others indicate that hormonal shifts upset circadian rhythms that control sleep patterns. Either way, insomnia is a primordial opening, a world inverted, where, as Elizabeth Bishop says, "left is always right, / when the shadows are really the body, / where we stay awake all night." In the dark I have the intimation of something coming closer, of a presence or the presence of a presence. "Here we go mother on the shipless ocean," the poet Anne Carson wrote. "Pity us, pity the ocean, here we go."

◎ ◎ ◎

My own night hunting is less like that of the owl that swoops from its perch and at the last moment extends its talons and closes its eyes, and more like the methodical nighttime work of the burying beetle. The burying beetle is black with scarlet scallops, and red tufts on the tips of its antennae. As night falls, the beetle is attracted to the smell of small dead snakes, birds, mice. On YouTube I watch as a beetle approaches a dead mouse, crawls underneath it, and lies on its back to push the body forward with its legs. Once a spot of soft earth is found, the beetle digs underneath the mouse, removes the fur, and works the corpse into an edible ball. "I shall have to frame that monstrous, infinite flesh," Clarice Lispector writes in *The Passion According to G.H.*, "and cut it into pieces that something the size of my mouth can take in."

On the last morning I took for granted that my mother was alive, I'd just bought my ticket at MoMA and was walking toward the galleries when my cell phone rang. It was my brother David, telling me that my mother's neighbor had called him to say newspapers were gathering on my mother's front porch. The neighbor had walked around to the back door, which was wide open to the elements, and called my mother's name. She did not answer.

While I was waiting for my brother to call me back to tell me what the police, who were on their way to the scene, found, I walked out of MoMA and up and down the New York City streets, past carts selling roasted peanuts and soft pretzels, tourists squinting into maps, and New Yorkers dashing to work. I was thinking she must be in the bathtub and was too embarrassed to call back. In my mind I sent out an SOS: *Are you OK?* I wandered into St. Patrick's Cathedral. There was a service going on so far from me it was as if I were watching people moving deep beneath the sea.

I continued to send out my signal. Finally an answer came: *I am safe.* I sat in the back pew, looking at the cross, the saint statues, a bank of electric votive candles. People talk about what a great comfort religion is during a crisis, but I felt the opposite. The symbols seemed ridiculous, like ancient broken toys. When my phone began to vibrate, I slipped out of the pew and the organ swelled and swept me out into the narthex, where my brother told me that my mother was dead.

I find it interesting that the voice I heard, or thought I heard, or in my misery imagined I heard, did not say *I am alive* but

I am safe. It's the kind of thing a person might say by text or cell phone once their flight has arrived in a foreign land: *I'm OK. I made it. I am on the other side.*

◎ ◎ ◎

Under the wedding photos, in the box of my mother's things, I find a composition notebook, mottled black and white, the same sort I have always used and am using now for my Flash Count Diary. I assume it's one of my own that my mother had saved from high school or college. But when I open the cover, I see not my messy handwriting but my mother's graceful cursive.

> *I was never loved, liked, appreciated. From the time I gave birth to Darcey he never loved me.*

> *I wanted to leave after Jonathan was born. No place to go—parents had no place for me and three kids.*

> *I was treated like dirt for 25 years and my willingness to lie down and be walked over allowed my kids to do the same to me.*

In the night, witness to her rage, I feel as I did in her presence. "I entered I knew not where," writes Saint John of the Cross. I feel sucked into a silence where my body is numb but my mind works frenetically.

———

What I have learned in the dark: (1) The devil, if he even exists, has nothing to do with it. (2) It's hard work to make something dead into food. (3) We have to make an absurd leap after horror has been revealed.

I waited in the car while my brothers went inside my mother's house. The coroner's office had taken my mother's body out earlier. The back of her house looked like the set of a horror movie. The small one-story cottage, the wood porch, the old-fashioned screen door. To the right of the porch, above a window-unit air-conditioner, I saw that a lamp was on in my mother's bedroom, illuminating a patch of wall and the darker indented corner. I imagined my brothers searching for the items we had talked about on the drive up: the safe-deposit box from the top shelf in the pantry, her jewelry box on her bedroom dresser, the papers in the plastic file folder on the attic stairs.

When the back door finally opened, I thought my mother was with my brothers, a dark shape floating just behind them as they locked the door and walked across the yard to the car.

At the hotel, my brothers and I drank whiskey straight from the bottle, and they told me of the chaos of the TV room. While she'd visited me at Christmas, no one had been inside her house since the fall. Much had changed since then. Piles of dirty clothes, trash, moldy dishes, empty containers, and newspapers were spread on the floor and soaked with urine.

Couch cushions stripped of their covers to the yellowed foam. "It was like a hamster cage," my brother said, and mentioned again that the back door had been wide open and that my mother's body had been found naked. Though the police were treating my mother's death as a natural one, my brothers and I were worried that someone had broken in, wrecked the house, maybe even assaulted my mother, causing what the coroner speculated was a heart attack.

In her journal, while blasting my father and us kids, my mother is mostly angry at herself. The fury she has for herself is the most violent. Why didn't she go to college after high school? Why did she get pregnant and marry my father? Why did she work at home and raise three children when neither my father nor we kids appreciated her? I think she even blamed herself for the divorce. *I made myself into a doormat.* She's mad at my father but also at how freely men move in the world. My father could have dealt better with my mother's misery, though I'm not sure anything any of us could have done would have changed her rage over how society treats older women. Several times in the journal she mentions the joke about trading in a forty-year-old wife for two twenty-year-olds.

My mother's story, the story of a mother and wife tossed at midlife to the sidelines, disconnected from a social network, barely able to support herself, is far from original. It's a story so familiar as to be outside of empathy, deactivated of its pain by repetition, by cliché.

The only entries in my mother's journals that look forward instead of back are the many about dieting. I know her weight was something she and my father fought over. Once when he asked me what he should get her for her birthday, I said chocolate. "I would never buy your mother candy," he said. Most of the dieting entries are procedural: *I can lose 1 pound every four days. I must lose 100 pounds.* And: *Fat makes Fat. Eat small portions.*

She often told me that fat was the last societally condoned prejudice. She understood the cultural cruelty, but her journal shows that she never stopped trying to get out from under the shame of being overweight. *I am all I have*, reads an entry in the last months of her life. *I must get healthy. It is not too late.*

● ● ●

Shame was the first feeling my mother had when she found out she was pregnant with me. And shame was her most insistent form of communication with me. Her father, my grandfather, drank, and her family never had much money. So even before I came into my mother's body, shame was like air to her, like water. It affected every aspect of her life, her perception of herself, her relationships, her ability to be intimate, her ability to take chances, to stick up for herself, to achieve in a career. Her shame didn't abate as she matured.

It increased: weight, menopause, divorce, breast cancer. After her mastectomy, on tamoxifen, her face got a shade of red closer to black, and she'd jump up and run to the window as if she'd actually caught fire.

Shame begins when a baby is seven months old. "That is the moment," the literary critic Eve Kosofsky Sedgwick has written in her book *Touching Feeling*, "when the mother's face, which mirrors the child's, refuses to play its part in the continuation of the mutual gaze, when for any one of many reasons it fails to be recognizable to the infant, and breaks the baby's faith in the continuity of the circuit." The child, no longer acknowledged and held inside the mother's gaze, feels abandoned, cast out. The baby concludes that it must have done something wrong and feels, for the first time, shame.

Even when I was an adult, my mother's face never lost its ability to unnerve me. As we watched *Elf*, I studied her features for signs of softening, any relaxation in the set of her mouth or the wrinkles in her brow. Her gray hair was held back with combs, and her face was pink and lovely. I looked into her eyes, not just for clues to her mood but also for the secret to myself. "In interrupting identity," Sedgwick writes, "shame makes identity. It's in the disconnection from the mother that the self in essence begins its life."

◉ ◉ ◉

Jung writes that in midlife we must find the corpse and bury it. The corpse being our former identity, the one we have outgrown and can no longer identify with. Once the corpse of our former life is buried, according to Jung, we float in a period of liminality, or what others have called the fertile void. During this time we have the chance, if we take it, to see ourselves more clearly. Simone Weil writes, "I am also other than what I imagine myself to be. To know this is forgiveness."

Rather than bury the corpse, my mother became the corpse herself. She was a pain devil, getting stiff and upset if my father's name was mentioned, raging about the unfairness of her own life and the sexist world in general. I looked to her for clues of what it was to be a woman, but what I saw was her powerlessness. "Many daughters," writes Adrienne Rich, "live in a rage at their mothers for having accepted, too readily and passively, 'whatever comes.'" For the first part of her life my mother was passive. She played the role of beauty queen, young mother, minister's wife. But after menopause, she no longer repressed her feelings. She raged, furious that men's freedom was absolute while her own was constrained.

◉ ◉ ◉

To combat my insomnia I have taken magnesium, which breaks through the blood-brain barrier. I have tried kava, hemp oil, valerian, melatonin, and a pill called Zen. I practice sleep hygiene: no screens after six, no eating after eight, New Age music, warm baths. I've listened nightly to a hypnotic CD on which a man with a soothing British accent tells me that sleep is delicious, encourages me to imagine person after person on a bus, lids heavy, heads drooping, till I'm the only one awake. I have, at the instruction of a Buddhist, not turned on any electric light and sat as twilight and then darkness fell. I got my doctor to prescribe doxepin, used to aid sleep.

The best remedy, though, remains meeting my mother in the dark, working, like the burying beetle, to make her body into food. Something I can ingest, take inside my body—a substance that will not poison but sustain me.

Last phone call: Out the window snow rushed down, flakes as big as potato chips and all the trees around covered in piles of white. After telling me about her dental problems, financial worries, and the newscaster who'd been accused of sexual harassment, my mother said, apropos of nothing: "You haven't always been kind to me." I started to defend myself for the zillionth time. "But in these last years," she interrupted me, "you have been kind."

My mother was an ambivalent feminist. She'd tell me that I should stop writing and stay at home with my daughter, Abbie. She told me she wished that rather than caring for me and my brothers she'd had a career. She despised elaborate second-marriage celebrations but once told me she wished she'd left my father earlier when it still might have been possible to build a life with someone else. With my mother there was always a paradox, an oppositional binary. That binary had to be healed in order to understand what she was trying to say.

When I wake in the dark, I often come back to that last night with my mother the day after Christmas. How she pulled out the photo of me in my wedding dress and pointed to where she thought I was exposed. Was she accusing me of being sleazy? Telling me that even on my wedding day I should feel shame? "Shame," Bernard Williams writes in his book *Shame and Necessity*, "is straightforwardly connected with nakedness, particularly in a sexual connection." The Greek word *aidos*, a derivative of the word for "shame," is a standard Greek term for the genitals.

In pointing to the photograph of me in my wedding dress, to the dark space between my legs, my mother was saying my body, like hers, was a female body and therefore an object of shame. Shame connected us, made us intimate. She was saying something upside down but true: showing me where I was implanted, growing inside her body on her own wedding day long ago, and implying that *she*, disguised as shame, was also inside me on mine.

◉ ◉ ◉

I'm almost to the bottom of my mother's box. I look through newspaper clippings of her beauty-queen years, mortgage papers for our house in Virginia, her baptismal candle. A white wax taper with the gold symbol for Alpha and Omega. There is a valentine from my dad, in which he has written a goofy love poem, as well as a letter from him after the divorce in which he demands the return of his favorite spatula.

You could read my mother's journal as the rants of a bitter, unhappy divorcée. Someone who blamed all her problems on others, my father in particular. You could discredit my mother's pain as familiar, trite. Her struggles and failures are so common they hardly delineate. But in another, more urgent reading, my mother's journal, like Margaret Atwood's *The Handmaid's Tale*, tells a story of a woman who was both humiliated and oppressed under patriarchy. A woman who nevertheless persisted, who stayed inside an active resistance even in her death.

My mother was on a slew of medications, none of which my brothers and I found. At first we suspected a home invader had taken them, but now I'm certain that weeks earlier she'd willfully thrown all her medicine bottles out. No one broke into my mother's house. She left the back door open, perhaps by accident but maybe because she knew she was in her last hours and didn't want us to have to break a window to get inside. I hope she left the door *open* in Rilke's sense of the word. An openness to something that comes from the strange, the other, the sacred, the new. The squalor of her room was not forced on her by an evil intruder but was of her own creation, or de-creation. A final fuck-you to the idea of soft-focus redemption.

In the dark I set my mother's baptismal candle into a brass holder and light a match. The taper throws out a circle of wobbling light. At the bottom of the box, underneath a stack of tax returns, I find a small notebook covered in red silk. Maybe it's her own flash count diary. But the pages inside are blank. How like my mother to save something so beautiful. When I closed down her house, I found brand-new sheets and comforters still in plastic, dresses with the tags still on, fancy soaps and lotions unused and at the back of the bathroom cabinet. In the attic, plastic containers filled with new pots and pans, a toaster, a teapot. I know many women of her age were in the habit of saving new things, though ten large plastic storage containers seem less like saving items for a current life than preparing for a hoped-for future one. Maybe I'm wrong, but I think my mother was saving each of those items as an act of rebellion as well as hope. My mother was waiting for a new world in which she'd have the dignity she knew she deserved, a world where she would not be invisible. The pages of the notebook are empty, but on the back flyleaf I do find my mother's voluptuous cursive.

Life is hard. Justice is as inconsistent as the people who create it. Accept this reality and continue to struggle or give up and lose control.

9 ● Hole in My Heart

I've come to the eleventh European Congress on Menopause at the RAI conference center in Amsterdam to learn how women in other countries are treated during the change. The congress pamphlet lists studies of the effects of black cohosh on women of Singapore, soy on Japanese women, flower extract on Korean women, and fennel cream on the women of Iran. I hope to learn about the association between sexual dysfunction and metabolic syndrome in the women of Turkey, the effect of vitamin D on bone strength in Brazilian women, and how hot flashes affect the work ability of the women in the Netherlands.

In the first hour I find that the results of these studies are not central to the congress but are simply displayed on posters in the back of the main atrium. The seminars and panels themselves focus on mainstream menopausal treatments. Case in point: a short Italian man in a blue suit with a labia-pink tie reports from the podium that even though there are not enough long-term studies, he believes hormones are the best treatment for the menopausal vagina. He talks of shrinkage, lack of pliability, dryness. All his descriptions explain how the vagina might feel to an incoming penis. The vagina as a viable penis holder. Not how a vagina might feel to the woman it belongs to.

After the panel, in the Q&A, a woman in a denim dress and flat leather sandals stands before the microphone. She introduces herself as a nurse practitioner and asks what the doctors think of the studies WHI, PEPI, and HERS, which show a risk of breast cancer, stroke, and dementia with extended hormone therapy. The doctors smirk at each other. The Italian tells the woman that if she'd actually read the studies, she'd see the risk is very small. He passes the microphone to the doctor beside him, who says, "If a woman wants to continue to have a sex life, she will need to do something about her vagina." The next questioner is a bald doctor in a blue cashmere sweater. He tells the panel he has been prescribing hormones in his practice for thirty years. "No wonder," the Italian jokes, "you look so young."

In her 1985 book *The Sex Which Is Not One*, the French feminist Luce Irigaray writes that female sexuality has always been conceptualized using male parameters: "The vagina is valued for the 'lodging' it offers the male organ. Understood in these terms, a woman's genitals never amount to anything but an envelope, a hole."

In the RAI lobby a salesman in wire-rim glasses demonstrates the MonaLisa Touch, in which a metal rod, laser-side up, is inserted into a menopausal vagina. A monitor on a pedestal nearby shows male hands covered in latex gloves inserting the rod slowly into the vulva, the labia folds. After the rod disappears inside the vulva, there is an animated sequence of the laser, like an elongated *Starship Enterprise*, flying in a roomy vaginal canal. Next a rose, that universal symbol of the female genitals. The rose's pink petals are wilted, hanging down, the edges brown. Through backward time-lapse photography, the petals get muscular, rise up around the stamen; they grow tighter and tighter until the rose is again a virginal bud.

"Heterosexual women's bodies are defined in relation to heterosexual male pleasure rather than their own pleasure," Virginia Braun writes in her 2010 essay "The Perfectible Vagina." In this definition, the tight vagina is fetishized. "The proper woman," writes Braun, "is constructed as childlike and virginal with an unused vagina."

Young women's vaginas are adored, fetishized. Menopausal vaginas ridiculed and medicalized. The vaginas of sex workers, something Amsterdam is famous for, are judged and reviled for the very quality men crave: their openness and availability. On the Internet I found a thread that compared experienced vaginas to a jar of mayonnaise, a large ziplock bag, a bucket of warm water, and the night itself. I learned that a woman's pussy is like a public restroom because it feels good but you wonder who else has been there. Vaginas, I learn, are much like screen doors—"The more they get slammed, the looser they get." Many jokes are addressed to prostitutes directly: "Ho, I'd kick you in the vagina but I don't want to lose my shoe."

The vagina in these jokes is a public space, a place where men meet, as in the one about a man who falls into a large vagina to find a number of other men, lost and searching for the exit. Even legally the vagina is constructed as a "thing," a space that can be searched. Alan Hyde, in his essay "The Legal Vagina," writes about a warrant that called for a search of the appellant's apartment and her vagina. "Law," Hyde writes, "constructs the vagina largely as a hiding place, full of secrets the eye cannot behold from outside, where drugs or other mysterious narratives lurk."

◎ ◎ ◎

Years ago my first husband told me, with deep reverence, about Amsterdam's window prostitutes. How cool they looked behind glass haloed in pink light. The night we arrived, in the late 1980s, it was after midnight as we searched for the houseboat hostel my first husband had stayed in during an earlier visit. We hunted canal to canal. By the time we gave up, all the hotels in our price range were full. One clerk told us he had a room separate from the hotel on the fifth floor of a nearby house. We followed the man across the street, up a narrow stairwell, and into a room that smelled of mildew, with a threadbare lavender bedspread and a lamp without a shade. The room was all dinge and shadow, like the hotel rooms in noir novels.

Even though it was late, my first husband wanted to go out walking. The canal water was black with shifting triangles of light, and the tall brick buildings with the gingerbread lattice looked like something off a Christmas card. We walked down a narrow alley called Bloedstraat, Blood Street. At first when I saw the red-light window, the woman standing in a black thong and bra, I thought something was wrong: a drunk girl outside a party must have taken off her dress. Close up, the woman looked placid and indifferent, like she'd just disrobed and was now standing in her bedroom doorway deciding what to do next.

"Let me introduce you," my first husband said, motioning to the woman in the window and making up names, "to Susan . . ."—he walked a few steps and pointed to the next window, behind which stood a woman in a black wig and white leotard—"and Carol." We walked farther down the street bracketed by a row of small pink-light windows. In each, like a monkey in a cage, was a woman for sale. My husband was excited, euphoric even; though no transaction would occur between himself and the women, he enjoyed feeling ownership over them, even if it was unrealized and hypothetical.

A mainstay of patriarchy is that there will always be, for a price, a hole open and ready for penetration. Here in De Wallen, this precept was not abstract but materially manifested. I realized the idea of the forever open and inviting hole was both a real space and a dream space and that, for my husband, its accessibility was one of the privileges of being a man.

Back in our room with the cigarette-scarred carpet and rust-stained bathroom sink, my husband pushed me down on the bed. He was aroused by the female bodies, the holes for sale, and frankly, in a creepy, abnegated, *Story of O* sort of way, so was I. After we both came, he fell asleep. I lay awake in the room watching the globe of a streetlight, like an alien force, shining through the thin curtains.

I'd learned about prostitution when I was eleven or twelve, just after I learned about sex. At first I was shocked, as all little girls are, to learn that the female body could be penetrated for cash. But eventually the fact became so normalized it seemed naive, even immature, to contemplate. In college, when I expressed my sadness over sex work, a man told me that I should see a shrink, that I was sexually uptight. Lying there in the dark hotel room, I was close to other female bodies. Bodies penetrable for a price. My husband was aroused by the open, available pussies, in part because his wife's pussy, my hole, was on a continuum, even interchangeable, with their own.

◎ ◎ ◎

In 1866 Gustave Courbet painted *L'origine du monde*, an image of a woman's sex up close, thighs spread, pink slit slightly open, surrounded by dark, generous pubic hair. The work, commissioned for Khalil Bey, an Ottoman diplomat and collector of erotic art, was kept behind a green velvet curtain Bey parted ceremoniously at late-night parties to entertain male guests.

Gambling debt forced Bey to sell the painting, which then fell into various hands. Looted by Russian troops in World War II, it was eventually brought back to Paris. In 1955, the French psychoanalyst Jacques Lacan bought the painting and hung it in his office in his country house in Guitrancourt. Lacan, who may be best known for his statement "Women do not exist," had his brother-in-law build a double frame with a wood panel cover for *L'origine*. "Lacan," Élisabeth Roudinesco writes in her book *Lacan: In Spite of Everything*, "loved to surprise visitors by carefully sliding back the panel to assert that Courbet was Lacanian *avant la lettre*: 'the phallus is in the painting.'" Lacan could not see the vagina but only the cock that had, to his mind, a moment before, pulled out.

● ● ●

The next day at the menopause conference in Amsterdam there is a luncheon underwritten by Fontana, a vaginal laser company whose machine is called SMOOTH. A panel of doctors praise the vaginal laser. "It pushes the clock back fifteen years," one doctor tells us. Another shares that when he first bought the machine for his practice he tried it out on his nurse. "After only one session," he says, "she got sexy with her husband."

Many of the online reviews for vaginal lasering are positive. Dozens of women, though, express disappointment: "No improvement after three treatments." Another woman is sore: "Not healing well and have a chemical burn. Why wasn't I warned of this side effect?" Most disturbing is the woman who, after her treatment, felt *vaginally traumatized*: "The laser hurt like a mother. It's a laser and it is inserted into your vagina and it resurfaces. In construction they call this sandblasting and that is what it felt like. I was gasping for breath and crying out, gripping the side of the table." When it was over, the woman, in shock, asked the nurse if her reaction had been normal, because nowhere had she read that the procedure would be painful. "Yes," the nurse said, "your reaction is normal."

I can understand that a tighter, smoother vagina might increase a woman's confidence in meeting male ideals. I remain unconvinced, though, that tightness and pliability are exclusively concerns of women. I worry too that vaginal rejuvenation may be a hoax. A year after the conference, in July 2018, the FDA sent warning letters to Cynosure, maker of the MonaLisa Touch, as well as six other laser companies, demanding that they stop claiming that their machines rejuvenated the vagina. "These products have serious risks and don't have adequate evidence to support their use for these purposes," said Dr. Scott Gottlieb, the FDA commissioner. "We are deeply concerned that women are being harmed."

Dr. David Matlock, the founder of the Laser Vaginal Rejuvenation Institute in Los Angeles and the star of the reality show *Dr. 90210*, is also famous for creating "a perfect wife" by giving his partner a surgical "Wonder Woman Makeover." On a 2010 episode of *The View*, Dr. Matlock holds up a plastic model of a vagina and explains that vaginal relaxation brought about by childbirth and aging is "a big, huge problem." To his patients, he peddles vaginal makeovers—an operation that could include labiaplasty, the cutting away of the labia; vaginoplasty, the cutting away and tightening of the muscles surrounding the vagina; and vaginal laser. *The View* host Joy Behar does not agree: "Don't you think this is a procedure that really makes men happy, not women?" Dr. Matlock shakes his head. When women come into his office, he says, he asks them if they want the vagina of an eighteen-, a sixteen-, or a fourteen-year-old girl. Whoopi Goldberg laughs uncomfortably, while Behar is clearly disgusted.

"If they say 'fourteen,'" Matlock continues, "I just shake my head and say, 'You bad, bad girl.'"

"We know," the feminist philosopher Jacqueline Rose writes, "that women are meant to look perfect, presenting a seamless image to the world so that the man, in that confrontation with difference, can avoid any comprehension of lack."

◎ ◎ ◎

In my small white hotel room on Spuistraat in the city center, I lie on my bed in my underwear and eat potato chips from the minibar and sip from a bottle of rosé. I watch seagulls out the window sweep over the tile roofs in the dimming purple light. The doctors at the conference are experts. They are supposed to know what is best for me. I wanted to believe them. But I didn't want to think of my vagina as failing, not normal, in need of immediate drug and laser intervention. Evolution ends my fertility and changes my body—it's natural. But this is not recognized. Instead the medical industry sees my body as deficient, an object to be fixed. I looked down at the loose skin of my thighs, the puddle of my belly, my veiny feet. Did they not understand how hard I was working to love my aging body? How hard I had to work to fight off disgust? "I was a body," writes Roxane Gay in her book *Hunger*, "one requiring repair, and there are many of us in this world, living in such utterly human bodies."

● ● ●

The psychoanalyst Ann Mankowitz feels that coming to terms with lost desirability is women's main menopausal challenge. "The problem of menopause," she writes, "is not that women no longer feel sexual desire, but that her ability to arouse sexual desire in others is waning." One of my menopausal correspondents agrees. "I remember," she said, "how men looked at me, talked about me, how I felt a certain power—it wasn't necessarily a sexual thing, but that was part of it. It was the power to ignite something complex that I could not completely understand."

Even my Buddhist friend who believes desire is the root of suffering, that detachment is the only avenue toward peace, does not want to lose her sexual desire, saying, "It's the main way I learn about myself." This is the friend who, when I have a crush, encourages me to, rather than act out, figure out what qualities my crush has—freedom, confidence, sensuality—that I want for myself. I don't disagree. A lover, consummated or not, can be a divine escort leading you to the beloved, the infinite, God.

In menopause the desire aimed at my body weakens, but my own desire has deepened, grown sophisticated, even metaphysical. Sometimes I feel I want God's body just as much as, if not more than, I do my husband's.

"Who is the real subject of most love poems?" writes the poet Anne Carson in her book *Eros the Bittersweet*. "Not the beloved. It is that hole." The hole as an emotional, as well as a physical, space. A lack. When I desire you, a part of me is gone.

"With this in mind," Georges Bataille writes in his book *Eroticism*, "we might say that sensuality is to mysticism as a clumsy try is to a perfect achievement."

◎ ◎ ◎

When it's completely dark I switch on the bedside lamp, pull on my jeans and T-shirt, and walk out of the hotel and into the Amsterdam night. The moon reflects in the dark water, a disk of broken silver that follows me canal to canal. The trees, in first bud, are blurry, delicate, sublime. I move *straat* to *straat*, and while it's not intentional I find myself once again in De Wallen, the red-light district.

I can't find Blood Street but I do find Gebed Zonder End, Prayer Without Ending street. I wonder if I've come to Amsterdam as much to revisit De Wallen as I have to attend the menopause conference. The area, though, is nearly unrecognizable from my earlier visit, with none of the low-fi seediness I remember. Now it's cranked. There seem to be as many storefronts selling vapable pot as selling sex.

Sex workers are dressed in outfits so outlandish they seem ironic. A woman in a floral bra and polka-dot stretch pants. Another wears a neon-yellow teddy and tall, tight rubber boots. With her white eyeliner and lipstick glowing under the black light, she looks like a moon goddess—Hecate or Kuhu, the one ancient people celebrated in festivals where they ate small crescent-shaped cakes. Back in the '60s, Amsterdam's red-light district storefronts were decorated like tiny bourgeoisie living rooms, with floral wallpaper, lamps, paintings, and curtains. Women, dressed like young wives, sat in upholstered chairs. These days sex is freed from domesticity. In just a handful of decades the sexual ideal has moved from a young wife in a sleeveless shift to women who look like characters in an anime cartoon: goddesses beamed down from a distant planet in a halo of green light.

◉ ◉ ◉

"Our woman with an open pussy" is how Duchamp referred to his final work, *Étant donnés*, in letters he wrote to his lover, the Brazilian sculptor Maria Martins. Critics have linked the work to Courbet's *L'origine du monde*, which Duchamp had seen reproductions of, as well as to *Woman in White Stockings*, another Courbet painting. In *White Stockings*, a nude woman sitting on the bank of a lake, with her sex facing the viewer, pulls a stocking over the toes of her extended right foot. The open pussy of Duchamp's nude, unlike Courbet's, is neither robust nor realistic but hairless, malformed.

Maria Martins, Duchamp's fifty-five-year-old lover, was the model for the female figure in *Étant donnés*. In 1946, at the most intense point of their secret affair, Duchamp cast Martins's body. A few years later, in 1950, Martins returned with her diplomat husband to Brazil, her native country. Duchamp felt as if he were *drowning*. "I feel totally lost," he wrote to her in a letter, "now that we are cut off from each other."

A stillness lies over *Étant donnés*: time has frozen, and the waterfall, the only living thing, is mesmerizing. The eye is drawn, almost magnetically, to the woman's genitals. There is no pubic hair, no vulva, no labia; just an off-centered slit leading into a strangely shaped hole. Critics have suggested that the sex is displayed in a rictus of death, that the work itself is a form of mourning for a lost and essentially dead lover. "Her muteness is compounded by our inability to remember her accurately," writes the art critic Helen Molesworth, "which is how I read the problem of the misplaced labia—as a physicalizing of the distortion of memory." Other critics have suggested the cunt is a frustrated mouth. Feminists have noted that the vulva is not abstract or unrealistic but traumatized. The woman has undergone a physical genital castration.

I have thought an inordinate amount about what, if anything, is wrong with the *Étant donnés* hole. Shaved pubic hair and vulva and labia that are at best shrunken and at worst cut away. Is Duchamp saying that the menopausal vagina is surreal? That a mature vagina, in its own way, is just as haunting as a virginal one? Maybe Duchamp is telling me that the cunts we see through peepholes, whether artistic or pornographic, are always dead. I wonder if he is mocking me, visually asserting that while the world is full of cocks, it has yet to come to terms with even one pussy.

The open pussy as *porte de sortie*, a kind of ultimate escape hatch. Each time a phallus enters a hole, there is the hope of material union, of bridging both a physical and a metaphysical gap. After the euphoria, though, often comes sadness. *Omne animal post coitum triste est.* "All animals are sad after sex." I found men in online chatrooms blaming women for this sadness: "If the girl is under what I would consider pretty, a 5 or less, my melancholy is fueled by a feeling of disgust at myself." "You get this depression if you've gone from banging a top shelf babe to a mediocre or poor quality girl." Disappointment, sadness, after sex, changes into hostility and falls, like a cement block, onto the female body.

◎ ◎ ◎

In one of the last conference sessions, doctors present case studies from their practices to a panel of experts. First up: Dr. Johannes Bitzer from Switzerland. A man in his late sixties, with a gray beard and rumpled sweater, he looks like

Freud the morning after a cocaine binge. Dr. Bitzer is different from the other doctors in his interest in holistic treatments for menopause: sex counseling, meditation, even light therapy. "A fifty-two-year-old woman," he begins, "comes in for her yearly checkup. At the end of the consultation, she says, 'I'm not interested in sex. If it would not be for my husband, I could live without sex, but I think it's a problem for him.'"

The first panel member, a thin man with a long, sallow face, grabs the microphone. He has many such cases in his practice. He says, "Husbands are getting Viagra and watching porn online for stimulation." He passes the microphone to the doctor beside him, who shrugs and says, "If his wife no longer excites him, what is to be done?" The final panel member, a tall Dutch doctor with a square jaw, leans into the microphone. His deep voice booms: "This couple is dysfunctional."

In literature, the most un-dysfunctional older couple I found was lesbian. In June Arnold's *Sister Gin*, the menopausal Su falls in love with the octogenarian Mamie Carter. In the novel's penultimate sex scene, Su finds that her lover's sex, while aged, is both erotic and compelling: "There was strength between [Mamie Carter's] legs and no dough there where the flesh was fluid enough to slip away from the bone and leave that tensed grain hard as granite and her upright violet part like an animal nose, against Su's palm."

Dr. Bitzer appears frustrated with the panel's response. No one has compassion for the woman's feelings or mentions exploring her desires. The audience, made up mostly of traditional doctors, suggests hormones, laser, anything to get the unworking vagina back into shape. "A lot of couples," Dr. Bitzer finally responds, "live dysfunctionally for decades." It is not a positive statement, but in its own way, it is the most empathetic thing I heard said at the eleventh European Congress on Menopause.

◎ ◎ ◎

"I'm not dead," the novelist Kathy Acker wrote. "I've got my cunt. I've got my cunt; it's not a hole; it's an animal and I love the animal."

10 ● The Whale Wins

The flight from JFK to Seattle is bumpy. I dig my fingernails into the skin of my thighs and promise God if she does not crash the plane, I'll be grateful, I'll finally accept that my life is not mundane but divine. After deplaning, I catch the Bellingham shuttle and ride several hours up the coast, stopping at, among other places, the Tulalip Casino, which sports a killer whale on its sign. At the Anacortes Ferry Terminal, I wait in a room—ticket window on one side, snack bar on the other—along with gray-haired people in casual clothing. Two young men, both with long ponytails. One wears a tie-dye T-shirt, the other a backpack. Three adorable little girls in matching Hello Kitty sweatshirts play around the feet of their mother, who wears a green sari with gold fringe.

———————

The Salish Sea is the home waters of J2, Granny, and all the other wild Southern Residents. It is this sea Lolita was taken from four decades ago. The Salish includes the water around the Strait of Georgia, the Strait of Juan de Fuca, and Seattle's Puget Sound. Two snowcapped mountain ranges, the Cascades and the Olympic, border Puget Sound. A multitude of rivers flow into the Salish, including the Columbia, Nooksack, Dungeness, and Chilliwack. On the ferry deck, wind rushes over my ears as I look out over the water, covered with silver light, moving the surface in one pattern, then another. A cormorant lands on the ferry rail near me. I see its iridescent purple neck, its black head and beak, and, when it opens its mouth, its blood-red throat.

● ● ●

In Friday Harbor, after I check in to my hotel, I walk across the street to Herb's, Friday Harbor's answer to *Moby-Dick*'s Spouter-Inn. Wood cutouts of killer whales hang from every streetlight, and in the gift-shop window I see killer whale cookie cutters, tea towels, skateboards, and oven mitts. The art gallery window displays killer whale wind chimes, mailboxes, and belt buckles. Inside Herb's there is no Melvillian wainscoting, no bulwark of an old-fashioned craft, no clam or fish chowder. Though the walls and ceiling of Herb's are covered in knotty pine that does give a feeling of being trapped beneath a capsized ship. From the ceiling hang a dozen orange life preservers. A school of carved-wood salmon swim, suspended, over the beer taps.

The inhabitants of Herb's are milder than Melville's half-wild sailors in their raggedy coats, heads muffled with woolen comforters, and beards stiff with icicles. While there are a few shaggy young men with impressive cases of bedhead who, I'll later learn, are kayak guides, the clientele at Herb's is mostly made up of sunbaked locals and weekend sailors. Only my bartender looks seaworthy, with his black beard, red handkerchief, and plethora of faded green tattoos.

Beside my beer lies the Center for Whale Research's *Matriline ID Guide*. I ordered the thick colored pamphlet, stapled at the spine, a year ago and already it's well-worn. Killer whale pods contain several matrilines, four generations of females, great-grandmothers all the way to great-granddaughters as well as sons. Each of the seventy-eight Southern Residents has a photo, a close-up of its dorsal fin and saddle patch. Every dorsal, which is located midway on the whale back, is shaped somewhat differently. All are triangular, but some are taller, others shorter; some bow at the top, others look like what Melville described as a "Roman nose." Many have nicks at the back of their dorsals from close encounters with boat propellers. The saddle patch is directly behind the dorsal, like a gigantic birthmark; each has a unique shape and color. Some resemble a cloud of wispy smoke; others are more white

than gray, as if snow had fallen onto the Salish Sea and settled on individual whales.

The killer whale body is huge, five times as long as a human's
and 150 times our weight. Their bodies are large but also
firm, muscular, and, to the human eye, wet, shining. Their
backs are black and stomachs white, and these opposing colors are in perfect unity, like a Chinese yin-yang symbol. Their
black pectoral fins jut from where the arms would be on a
land mammal, like two flat paddles. Their tail flukes, mis-
taken for mermaid tails by early sailors, are bow shaped, indented in the middle. Just in front of their white oval eye
patches are the small eyes, which, like human eyes, can be
either brown or blue. Killer whale snouts, where a nose would
be, narrow like a dolphin's. Inside their pink mouths, their
tongues are the size of a bath towel, and they have rows of
large top and bottom teeth. Blowholes are located on the
top of the head, a hollow opening the size of a cantaloupe
covered with a flap of black skin that closes while they dive
underwater. Killer whales, unlike humans, who breathe un-
consciously, are conscious breathers. They must, when they
need oxygen, rise to the surface, open the blowhole flap, ex-
pel a smelly gust of wet air, and suck in a new breath.

I'd hoped to memorize the dorsals. I'm particularly interested
in the matriarchs. J16, a whale known as Slick who was
born in 1972, has a classic dorsal with a saddle patch that
looks like a roiling storm front. K12, also born in 1972, and

known as Sequin, has a thick, squat dorsal and a faint, lacy saddle. L25, the eighty-five-year-old whale thought to be Lolita's mother, has a straight dorsal with just the slightest top curve and a gauzy white saddle. I realize as I stare down at the pages of the *Matriline ID Guide* that it's impossible: I will never be able to tell one whale from another. I won't get close enough to see their saddle patches, and to my untrained eye, all the dorsals will look similar. I decide to concentrate on J2, Granny. Her dorsal is wide, with a large indentation in the center. The nick, probably from a boat propeller, is more curved than triangular. J2's saddle itself is shaped like a small killer whale calf.

I've learned as much as I could about Granny. She was born in 1911, the same year as both Ginger Rogers and Mahalia Jackson. She was once seen with her pod as they drove transient whales that dared to hunt in J pod territory up onto the beach. In 2011 Granny started to travel with J37, Hy'Shaque. About a year later, when J37 had her first calf, some speculated that Granny may have been giving the new mother advice. Since then she is often seen near her great-grandson L87, a twenty-five-year-old whale who recently lost his mother. Granny's been spotted playing with porpoises and babysitting younger members of her pod so their mothers could forage. Dr. Deborah Giles, the former director of research for the Center for Whale Research and the current resident scientist at the Friday Harbor Labs, told me that many times she'd seen J pod swimming down Haro Strait, with J2 slapping her tail flukes "like a schoolteacher blowing her whistle." Quickly, not only J pod but also K and L pods would line up behind.

While J2 is the most iconic female, J1, who was thought to be Granny's son and known as Ruffles, was the most iconic male until he died in 2011. Ruffles was easily recognizable from his huge wavy dorsal fin and the slow, deliberate way he dived. Known to whale scientists as "the big guy," J1 loved to surf. "He'd make a beeline for the container ships," Dr. Giles told me, "and bodysurf in the wake off their stern." Younger male whales forage for the day in groups but at night return to their mother's side. Relationships between matriarchs like Granny and their male sons are close. Older mothers catch salmon for their male offspring. The mother-son relationship is so crucial that when a mother dies, her son is eight times more likely to die in the year after. This could be because of the loss of food, but Dr. Giles speculates it could also be emotional: "While females have calves to care for, male whales' main emotional bond throughout their lives is with their moms." J1 while alive was "glued to" J2's side. He was also the guardian of the greater pod. Once when J pod came up to a whale-watching boat, it was J1 who stayed the longest, making sure J42, the newborn Echo, and his mother, J16, known as Slick, were safely past the boat propeller before he swam off behind them.

Each whale has its own personality, its own physicality, and its own part in whale culture. Whales, like humans, have both vertical and horizontal culture. "Culture," as Hal Whitehead and Luke Rendell write in their 2015 book, *The Cultural Lives of Whales and Dolphins*, "is a flow of information from one animal to another." Vertical culture, the historical skills passed down from generation to generation, includes language, foraging techniques, and sexual and social behavior. Transient whales teach their calves to beach themselves, catch a seal, and then refloat back into a receding wave. Mothers have been seen on sealless beaches, teaching their calves this skill. The Southern Residents' greeting ceremony is also learned. Each pod forms a long line, then after a moment of silence, K, L, and J pods begin to vocalize loudly and break into tight subgroups with their friends in other pods. This ritual, like square dancing or a religious ceremony, is taught by older pod members to younger ones.

Horizontal culture is a fad, something that develops quickly, catches on, and then passes through the community fast. Think pixie haircuts, Rollerblades, ant farms. The biggest fad to swerve through the Southern Resident community was in 1987. That summer, a female in K pod began to push around and play with a dead salmon. Within five weeks, nearly every member of K, L, and J pods had a dead salmon toy. By fall, though, the whales lost interest, and not one was seen pushing or carrying a dead salmon on its snout.

Language is the most important part of cultural transference. Killer whales make a rich variety of echolocation clicks and calls. The calls follow different patterns and are a communication system similar to Morse code. Each pod has more than a hundred calls. Some of them are shared by all the pods; others are unique to individual pods. The whales produce sounds by forcing air through various nasal sacs and cavities; the sounds reverberate up through the whale's fatty forehead and are beamed out acoustically like a ray of sonar.

Erich Hoyt, one of the first people to study whale language in the 1970s, recorded whale calls, then tried, by slowing down the notes, to replicate them on his synthesizer. He reports that on one boat trip with a film crew, several whales became fascinated with the underwater hydrophone attached to the bottom of the boat. They directed a series of tense vocalizations toward the hydrophone. Hoyt flipped on the tape recorder, turned up the volume pots on the synthesizer, and pressed the keys in the pattern that mimicked the calls. "Two seconds went by," Hoyt writes, "and then it came: A chorus of whales—three, maybe four—sang out a clear, perfect imitation of what I had just played to them." What astounded Hoyt was that rather than making their original call, the whales duplicated Hoyt's slower, stilted human version.

Sex is also an important and frequent part of whale life. "The whales are very tactile," Giles tells me, "very sensuous." Groups of young males have been seen playing together with their penises, known as sea snakes—six feet long and as thick as a fire hose—draped over one another. Mature males find breeding partners in other pods. The matriarchs, like killer whales in general, appreciate sexual pleasure and seek it out. "It was not unusual to see sex play going on," Giles tells me, "and see that J2 was in the mix." Older females may train the younger males in sexual technique. They may use sex to relieve tension in their pods, or they may just like sex. "In their culture," Giles says, "they don't have that human taboo: don't sleep with old women."

When sex does lead to procreation, whale birth is a communal affair. After a female whale gives birth, multiple females, including matriarchs, gather around the newborn and lift it up to the surface for its first breath. "There are so many females," the whale scientist Alexander Morton wrote, "there is no telling who the mother was, they touch the baby all over." The tooth marks on the head of J50 when she was born may mean that the baby was breech and that an older female, maybe even Granny, served as midwife, pulling the calf out of the mother.

◉ ◉ ◉

I'm the first to arrive at the Friday Harbor traffic circle, in front of the ferry dock, where I'm supposed to meet the van that will take me whale-watching. I sit on a bench and read *The Unprofessionals*, a 2008 novel by Julie Hecht that features a menopausal narrator: "It was the second month of living without a soul and I was getting used to the feeling. The obliteration of the self had begun two years before—probably it had begun many years before—but now I was at the brink of being seriously over forty-nine and it was all coming to fruition."

At Smallpox Bay, which has a black stone beach and empties into Haro Strait, we park the van, unload the kayaks, and carry them down to the beach. The guides—Matt, a college student with long red hair held back in a ponytail; and Will, a recent graduate from Michigan's Upper Peninsula—tell us how to wear our life preservers, put on the spray skirt, hold our paddle, and feather the blade sideways if we're taking a break. Beside me there is a young couple: the man, after being asked if he likes whales, turns around and pulls up his shirt to show off his humpback tattoo. Another couple, in expensive gear, works at Animal Planet. The only other single person is a woman near my own age, a Broadway producer. She has dyed-black hair and tight, pale skin. We compare gear, our Gore-Tex jackets and neoprene shoes. Matt tells us never to stand up in the kayak. He demonstrates the straddle-butt drop, and side swing-in. Will explains that if we see whales, we'll quickly do what is called "rafting up": pull our boats close together and hold on to each other's paddles. This way we are less likely to tip over.

I'm in front and Matt is in back as we push out, stern first, into the shallow water. An egret grasps a silver fish and tips its head back so that the fish slips inside its beak and down its long neck. Out in the bay the water is rougher. I'm surprised how low the kayak sits in the water, how the boat shifts and bumps on every swell. We paddle toward Lime Kiln Light-house, home of the hydrophone I've been listening to for months. Matt points out an eagle's nest high up in a pine tree and the eagle itself, sitting in the top branches of the crooked, red-barked madrone tree. The colors are divergent: yellow grass, red bark, the deep green leaves, and then the water, which is slate blue with swatches of viridian.

Will points out a fried-egg jellyfish, translucent pale blue with a yolk-like center. Purple stars cling to rocks below the tide line. We rest in a patch of bull kelp, each plant like a giant scallion with a large glassy bulb and long flat stems floating underneath. Matt tells us about the seals we see ly-ing out on the rocks, chunks of fat covered in sleek fur. I'm beginning to understand that rather than being a whale-watching trip, this is more of a nature tour. When we paddle back into the bay for our lunch break, it's clear we're not going to see whales. I eat my energy bar and put on my sun-glasses to hide my disappointment.

The graduate student who watched the 751 hours of whale footage—the basis for the whale menopause study—got in-terested in the Southern Residents while working as an in-tern at the Center for Whale Research on San Juan Island. "They each had their own personality," Emma Foster told me. "Some are playful, others shy." Foster spent her week-days watching whales on the center's boat and found herself drawn, even on her days off, to Lime Kiln Point State Park, where she watched for whales from shore. "It's the most amazing feeling seeing them," she said, "very addictive and very strange." Unlike me, Foster memorized the dorsals and saddle patches of all the Southern Residents. What she learned from watching the footage, taken over fifteen years, was that in times of food scarcity, when the salmon supply was low, it was the oldest post-reproductive females that led their pods.

After lunch we load back into the kayaks. The wind is less severe now, the water placid. Smooth. As we clear the bay mouth and move out into the Salish Sea, the guy with the humpback tattoo says he thinks he sees whales to the west. I see them, small black-and-white shapes, breaching and spyhopping. Matt has us raft up. I grip my neighbor's paddle. Will holds on to the bull kelp, rooted in the seafloor, so we don't drift. Matt says if there were more time he'd tuck us into a nearby cove. The whales are moving fast, making their serpentine way in and out of the water. Their dorsal fins are bigger than I imagined, towering over the sea. Massive heads push giant pillows of rippled water in front of them. Each time they rise, breaking the surface, the sea streams off their backs like rainwater sheeting off a tilted roof. The theater lady is worried they are swimming directly at us. Could we capsize? Matt reminds us to hold each other's paddles tight. I feel the kayak rise up a little in the water.

As the whales swim closer, talking stops. The concentration is acute, singular. I feel my pulse speed up, my heart shaking my rib cage. Two whales surface ten feet in front of our kayak, their eye patches so white they glow and their dorsal fins stretching high in the air. *Kawouf!* Their blowholes go off one after another. The kayaks jumble together on the confused sea. I am a small land creature floating on the edge of a vast ocean populated by giants. When I look down, I see several whales swimming beneath our boats, white tummies moving under translucent green water. Our kayak rises up and in front of me, only a few feet away, is a massive killer whale. *Kawouf!* I see a brown eye looking directly at me, the shining, numinous expanse of body. "It's Granny," Matt says. "I see the notch."

In the van on the way back, silence continues. I feel blissed-out, sleepy. When I get back to my hotel room, I call up people on the East Coast to tell them I've seen Granny. I feel a strong need to share. But each time I tell the story of the huge black-and-white creatures surrounding our raft of yellow kayaks, I feel, after I put down the phone, a sense of loss, of somehow selling out the experience, making the encounter sound like yet another entertainment. When I describe the whales as vibrant, muscular, huge, the whales become visual objects separate from myself. But what I actually felt was a dilation.

I'd later learn what I'd experienced is known by local boat captains and naturalists as an orca-gasm. "When the whales surface, people first get quiet," one guide tells me. "Then they make sex sounds, heavy breathing, aahs, oohs, and 'oh my god.'" Seeing whales is not passive but an embodied experience. "When the whales breach," one park ranger told a researcher, "it's like a climax. People don't get this way about foxes."

I have trouble falling asleep that night. There is the usual menopausal sleeplessness. It is stuffy, my room has no air-conditioning to combat Washington State's rare heat wave, and I can hear music coming out of Herb's across the street. Whenever anyone leaves or enters, noise flares out. Mostly I am still high off seeing Granny. J2 is a holy, mythological beast, one who gave off a powerful charge.

This was not a warm, fuzzy feeling. "One does not meet oneself," the naturalist Loren Eiseley has written, "until one catches the reflection from an eye other than human." Granny's eye was watchful, removed, judicious, and uneasy. "The animal looks at us," Derrida writes, "and we are naked before it. Thinking perhaps begins there."

For years I'd been reading the transcendentalists, those lovable Victorian hippies. I'd read Emerson's essay "Nature" slowly, stopping to meditate on favorite passages: "Nature will bear the closest inspection. She invites us to lay our eye level with her smallest leaf and take an insect view of its plain." I wanted, as the transcendentalists had, to feel the divine in nature. "Nature," Thoreau writes, "is full of genius, full of the divinity; so that not a snowflake escapes its fashioning hand." Now I was realizing that nature was not *full* of divinity, that the transcendentalists had not gone far enough. *Nature itself was divinity.* Galway Kinnell writes, "If the things and creatures that live on earth don't possess mystery, there isn't any."

As a minister's daughter, I have always thought a lot about the spiritual realm. I'm continually reading books on the roots of Christianity, Sufi cults, and Buddhist masters. I make retreats to monasteries and listen to theological podcasts. None of this makes me spiritually smarter. Actually I'm sort of dense when it comes to religion. Faith is not natural to me. Confronted by the whale, much of my theology seemed speculative, even flimsy. I want both the "more" that William James writes about but also the "real" that J2 engenders.

When I wake later, the music has stopped. I look out my window at the textured glass shade of the streetlight, the bright edge of a building, one window's inky shine. I know I should sleep, but my new position in the universe is making my brain feel as if it is on fire. And not because of hormonal withdrawal. I don't want time to keep going forward, separating me from the whales, from Granny. I felt a little as I had the night after my daughter was born. After pushing out a creature wet with saltwater and blood, I felt at life's oceanic center. Every minute moving forward separated me from an experience too big to absorb. It was a real thing, though it could not be represented as value but only, as the philosopher Jean-Luc Marion explained, as the "impossible," like birth, death, eros, God. Seeing J2 was like having my daughter, an event outside human evaluation.

◉ ◉ ◉

The transport plan for freeing Lolita from her tourist-trap captivity in Miami reads like a science fiction novel. Lolita will be lifted by crane in a sling specifically made for her massive body. The pectoral fin cutouts will be lined with "anti-rubbing fabric." On the cargo plane, preferably a Boeing C-17 Globemaster, her tank will be kept cool with ice cubes. The team of vets and trainers who will go along with her, all in matching wet suits, will repeatedly spread moisturizer on her dorsal fin, as well as spray her with water. Using a suction cup, vets will continuously monitor Lolita's heart.

Once Lolita's plane touches down in Seattle, she will be renamed Tokita, the original Salish name given to her by the veterinarian who selected her out of Puget Sound for the Seaquarium. She will be transported by truck and ferry to Orca Island. Once in her sea pen, Lolita will be trained to disassociate humans from feeding. She will learn to forage for live salmon. Within time, L pod, which includes both her mother, L25—Ocean Sun—and three other members of her pod that witnessed her brutal 1970 capture, will swim near enough for Lolita to hear their vocalizations. The hope is that Lolita will respond, which would bring L pod closer. "The reunion to follow," reads the Orca Network release document, "would be an unprecedented event in the collective memory of Lolita and her family."

When I first learned of Lolita's captivity and the plan to set her free, I assumed she'd be released in a matter of months. Protesters turn dozens of cars away from the Seaquarium every Saturday and Sunday, and negative press is longstanding and persistent. Many times I fantasized of being near the sea pen, on Orca Island, when Lolita was lowered into her home waters. But though animal advocates continue to protest and litigate for her release, I see now that the Seaquarium will never release Lolita. The company that owns the Seaquarium, Palace Entertainment, also owns Boomers Long Island, Story Land, Dutch Wonderland, and a place called Wet 'n Wild, as well as fifty other amusement parks. In 2007 Palace Entertainment was sold to the Spanish company Parques Reunidos for $330 million. On its investors' webpage, the company reports that after a dip in 2015, attendance at all its parks is now on the rise. Earnings for 2016 were more than $584 million.

◉ ◉ ◉

Lolita, if free, could be a post-reproductive pod leader, one of the matriarchs whose leadership is helping scientists understand why menopause has evolved. According to Darwinian fitness, a creature will continue to breed until it dies, having as many offspring as possible. Menopause, with its midlife cessation of fertility, goes against this most powerful of precepts. There are a number of theories that try to explain why menopause developed. Extended longevity was the first and is still the most pervasive theory—the idea that we simply outlive our fertility, that menopause exists only because we should be dead. Proponents of this theory argue that in earlier times women did not live much past their fifties. But new research has shown that high infant-mortality rates skewed statistics and that there has always been a portion of women who lived well past menopause. The theory of reproductive conflict proposes that rather than compete with our adult daughters, we lose the ability to reproduce. Our energies, according to this theory, are better spent supporting our daughters' fertility than competing with it. Mate choice theory claims that because all men, younger and older, prefer younger women, older women eventually evolved out of reproducing. Mate choice has been heavily disputed, because while men claim to prefer younger partners, many primates, including chimpanzees, prefer older ones.

I've renamed the patriarch hypothesis, championed by Harvard's Frank Marlowe, the Hugh Hefner hypothesis. This theory proposes that once males become capable of maintaining high status and reproductive access beyond their prime, selection favors the extension of maximum life span. The longevity gene is not on the Y male chromosome but on the X female one. In other words, we are dragged along into menopause and beyond because men began to live longer to fuck younger women: "As his mate reached menopause, a male tried to acquire a younger female, and the higher-status males succeeded in doing so. Selection then favored even greater longevity in males who could double their fitness by starting a second family with a new wife."

As you might have guessed, all the above theories were both discovered by and propagated by men, and were tested mostly using computer simulation and game theory. Kristen Hawkes, the expander of the grandmother hypothesis, based her research on living tribes of hunters and gatherers. In the 1980s, Hawkes studied the Aché, a group of nomadic hunters and gatherers in Paraguay. It was there she noticed that the men of the tribe were not providing enough food for their families: "The meat from the hunt was divided between all in a community and was also sporadic." Hawkes went on to study the Hadza hunters and gatherers in Tanzania. There she began to figure out how families got the food they needed: "They were right in front of us. These old ladies who were just dynamos. Women in their sixties and seventies bringing in as much or more food—tubers and berries—for their families as younger women." The grandmother hypothesis states that older women stop having babies at midlife so they can be free to provide for their daughters' offspring and also advise the community at large. "You can't really call women who are past their childbearing years post-reproductive," Hawkes says, "because while they may not be fertile, there is a lot of evidence that they are doing important things for the reproduction of their genes."

"I find it fascinating," Darren Croft, a professor of animal behavior at the University of Exeter, told me, "that the same reproductive strategy evolved in both humans and killer whales." Croft calls menopause "a big evolutionary puzzle." His killer whale research, along with that of Emma Foster, showed the worth of post-reproductive pod leaders: "The oldest and most experienced individuals were those most likely to know when and where to find food." Just as in the whale pods, older women were "key in hunter-gatherer communities." These individuals can improve the ability of groups to solve problems and respond to potential dangers. This transfer of information is the key to the selection of menopause. "It's amazing," Croft told me, "how much the whales tell us about ourselves."

● ● ●

After I see J2, Granny, leading her pod up Haro Strait, I assume I'll see whales again a few days later on my three-day camping trip. This time my guide is Sam, a serious young man with hazel eyes and ginger hair and beard. Our group includes a doctor couple from Colorado, both CrossFit champions in their over-seventy age group; a scientist who studies bees; and her partner, a French expert on artificial intelligence. Then there is Wayne, an Ohio prison guard, and his daughter Vickie, a competitive cheerleader. As we gear up and pack the kayaks, Vickie, who is wearing a SAVE THE WHALES T-shirt and an orca necklace and earrings, takes frequent selfies of herself smiling.

We paddle nearly four hours, ten miles over wild, roiling water into Reid Harbor to Stuart Island, a campsite once used as a Salish summer residence. The trees soar around a dozen campsites and a raised clapboard outhouse. The bay scintillates in the dimming sunlight. I set up my tent, roll out my sleeping bag. I listen to Wayne and the doctors talk outside my tent about Jesus. The male doctor, who is an obstetrician, says that whenever he delivers a baby, he feels the presence and glory of Jesus. *Why Jesus?* I write in the little notebook I pull out of my dry bag. Why not the wonders and glory of the female body?

At the picnic table in the middle of our campsite I chop vegetables for our dinner while Sam sets up the propane stove. He tells me about the program he just came from in Panama where he studied pygmy sloths and the Ph.D. program in ecological behavior and evolution he'll attend at U.C. San Diego in the fall. He works efficiently, unpacking the plastic tubs of cooking supplies, fry pan, jar of salsa, tin plates, and blue enamel coffee mugs. Vickie comes over. She tells us she got interested in orcas by watching the film *Free Willy*. For a while she played the SeaWorld live-cam day and night. After she saw the film *Blackfish*, she realized captivity was wrong. This trip to see the whales, a trip Vickie's father has saved up for, is a high school graduation present.

After dinner, while everyone is sitting around the campfire, Wayne corners me on my way back from the outhouse.

He heard me say that my father was a minister, that I teach college, and that I have a complicated relationship with faith. Wayne tells me he has a video he wants to send me. In it, a former Stanford professor talks about how his education made it hard for him to accept Jesus. "Once the professor put that aside," Wayne tells me, "he and Jesus could be friends."

Do I want to be friends with Jesus? I've certainly spent a lot of time thinking about him, even being jealous of his singular connection to the divine. At the moment, if I was forced to pick a Jesus story, it would be the one about the woman with the flow of blood in the book of Mark. Also known in Greek as *haemorrhoissa*, "bleeding woman." Various translations list the blood flow as discharge, hemorrhaging, and—my favorite—flux. The woman with a flux of blood. This woman has lived for years in a constant state of uncleanness, according to Jewish law. This woman touches the fringe of Jesus's robe. She doesn't need his hands to rest on her head or to feel the warmth of his caress. The bleeding woman's own agency stops the flow of blood. She does not need to befriend Jesus in order to be made whole.

On the second day, as we paddle from Stuart to Posey Island, Sam tells us about the challenges faced by the endangered Southern Residents. Noise pollution both stresses the whales out and makes it hard for them to forage and navigate. Pollution. Toxins, including PCBs collected in female killer whales, are off-loaded in breast milk, making survival rates of calves extremely low. Food scarcity. Salmon are diminishing both in number and size. Reasons for this include overfishing, dams that block natural spawning patterns, and disease. Wild salmon break into coastal sea pens, where salmon are farmed, and catch infestations, most commonly flesheating lice. A recent scientific report, Sam tells us, speculates that in one hundred years, if salmon scarcity continues, the Southern Residents will become extinct.

"Like the others," writes W. S. Merwin in his poem "The Last One," "the last one fell into its shadow. / It fell into its shadow on the water. / They took it away its shadow stayed on the water."

Posey Island, at the mouth of Roche Harbor, is tiny. Just big enough for a half dozen campsites and an outhouse. The coastline is jagged black rock. Seals, like small bald men, swim by. It's cold, overcast. Vickie is grumpy because we haven't seen orcas. I've pitched my tent on the other side of the island, away from the others, and after dinner, around sunset, Sam comes around and sits out on the rocks. He's frustrated. The hardest part of his job is managing people's expectations about seeing whales. People have asked him, *When do you let the whales out?*—as if the Salish Sea were one big SeaWorld. They've said sadly, *We only saw a humpback.* Some want their money back if no whales are spotted. What frustrates him most is when people see the whales and are still disappointed. "People," he tells me, "have lost the ability to understand the concept of wild."

Sam asks, since he knows I've read a dozen books on cetaceans, if I think the whales have spiritual lives. I tell him about the sun ritual in Alexander Morton's book *Listening to Whales: What the Orcas Have Taught Us*. Morton worked in the 1970s with the SeaWorld orcas Corky and Orky. Every morning before the sun rose, the two whales squirted water at a spot where the water met the tank wall. Morton writes, "They licked that spot with their thick pink tongues and spy-hopped next to it." As the sun rose, the first ray of light crept down the tank side and touched the water in the exact spot the whales had marked. "Through the months the spot moved in response to the earth's rotation, but the whales always knew just where the first shaft of light would hit the water." Sam tells a story, relayed to him by another guide, of seeing a killer whale mother carrying her dead calf around on her rostrum. Eventually she tried to wedge the dead baby into a crevice in the shoreline rock, much like a pallbearer might place a coffin inside a mausoleum.

That night at the campfire, two groups emerge. Wayne, Vickie, and the doctors are talking again about Jesus, his extreme suffering, how lucky we are to have someone who suffered like that for us. This makes me crazy. First of all, why would you want someone to suffer for you? Second, every single day, as well as throughout history, there are people who suffer as much as if not more than Jesus. The other group consists of Sam and the scientist couple. Their conversation centers around new DNA testing, how it's delineating new species. A western blackbird species has now been discovered to be two separate species. Neither conversation holds me. I drift down the path to the other side of the island, where my tent is pitched. I lie down inside my sleeping bag, prop my head up on my backpack, and look out at the silvered water. The stars are myriad, like salt spilled on violet paper. My arms ache from the hours of paddling, and I still feel, like after a long car trip, that I'm moving, gliding over the rolling water, both at odds and at one with the sea.

In the morning we break camp. Vickie asks Sam when we will see whales. Sam is sheepish, telling her he heard on the short-wave radio that J pod had been seen in Haro Strait. The whole way back home to Smallpox Bay, around Henry Island, past Mosquito Pass, and back into Haro Strait, as I paddle, the wind is in my face, pushing my hair back, making it impossible to hear anything anyone says. The current is behind us, but it does not feel like it. The waves are tall, and each time the tip of our kayak flaps down, I'm pelted with a sharp spray of saltwater.

After we've unloaded the kayaks and stored the gear in the van, we eat lunch on a bluff over Smallpox Bay. Vickie sits away from the group on a metal bench, her face turned in profile toward the sea, her arms folded across her chest and her forehead bunched. When her father joins her, she shrugs off his arm and runs down the path back toward the van. The rest of us look at one another; the Colorado doctors are seasoned campers, enthusiastic about the trip, whales or no whales, and the scientists understand that animals will not show themselves on a human schedule.

Wayne and Vickie sit in the back of the van weeping. Wayne holds his hand over his face and Vickie's shoulders shake; it's a forlorn misery, as if they've been abandoned by their savior. I'm the first, beside them, back in the van. I'd like to separate myself from Vickie, but I am also a whale-watching pilgrim, vulnerable and seeking. I flew across the country; took a shuttle, then a ferry; and finally climbed into a kayak in order to get close to the whales. I dreamt of an audience with the great matriarch J2 and I was not denied. If I had not seen Granny, I too would have wept.

All trip, Wayne has been pressing his theology on me. Now I offer a bit of my own. "Whales are like God," I say. "Not seeing them is just as important as seeing them." They both look at me, not at my face but at the space just above my head, like babies do. "Here is the great difficulty," Alan Watts writes, "in passing from the symbol and the idea of God and into God himself. It is that God is pure life, and we are terrified of such life because we cannot hold it or possess it, and we will not know what it will do to us."

––––––––

The Leviathan, the whale, above all other creatures, is a stand-in for God. A placeholder. Ahab loses his life in trying to control the white whale. After Jonah refuses to obey divine instruction, God sends the whale to swallow him. The verbs used to connote God's relationship with the whale vary according to biblical translation. On BibleGateway.com, I consider the various versions. In the English Standard, God *appointed* the whale, as if God were an upper-level manager moving his creature to a new post. In the International Version, God *provided* the whale: God as the ultimate prop master. The Lord *prepared* the whale in the King James Version: God as film director working with a difficult Method actor. *Prepared* is clearest. God trains his divine emissary to do his bidding. Still, the accuracy is off. God and whale are not separate but one. I offer my own crude translation: God, the whale, swallowed me.

● ● ●

Back in Brooklyn I have a dream that I'm sitting in a cavernous room, writing at a small desk, like the IKEA one I use upstate. Far above my head in a corner I see books, volumes lined up according to subject. I am in a library. My desk shifts, the legs sinking into plush pink carpet. I scribble words on a legal pad. After a while I look up again. I see a line of emaciated stone saints. I am in a cathedral, not a library. I write some more. It's the third time I look up that I see the gigantic, rounded rib bones and, above my head, the long and elegant spine.

11 ● Home Waters

The low point of my second trip to the San Juan Islands came on the last night of camping. This was on Stuart Island, a location that in the rain had lost much of last summer's charm. My fellow campers this time were a group of engineers, men in their sixties with their adult sons. In the kayak I was paired with one of the sons, a young robotics expert who nagged me to paddle harder and talked relentlessly of driverless cars run by robots. When I told him about writing this book, he asked incredulously what whales could possibly have to do with menopause. It didn't help that my beloved J2, Granny, was dead. In October 2016, just a few months after I'd seen her, she was reported missing, and by the end of the year, listed as deceased.

———

I wasn't in the San Juans in late December 2016 when the Center for Whale Research changed Granny's status from missing to dead. "Everybody was saddened," Friday Harbor's mayor, Farhad Ghatan, told me. "It was quiet around town." Businesses put R.I.P. GRANNY signs in their windows, and the Whale Museum had a community potluck where locals told stories of encounters with the matriarch. Dr. Giles stressed the expanse of J2's life, all the changes she lived through. She saw salmon decrease not only in number but also in size, shrinking from one hundred pounds apiece to barely twenty. Salmon got smaller while boats got bigger; mammoth cargo ships now move back and forth down the Strait of Juan de Fuca. She lived through all the marine park captures, witnessing not only calves like Lolita being taken out of the water in canvas slings but also five whales drowning as they struggled in the nets.

Through all these traumas and changes, Granny remained a versatile and empathetic leader. "When you have a problem," one of the postmenopausal women I interviewed told me about her Caribbean American culture, "it's the matriarch you go to." Granny was sometimes seen swimming alongside a younger member of her pod. Other times she was alone, as if in contemplation. Most often J2 was seen out front leading not only J pod but also K and L pods as well. "She was a charismatic leader," Giles says. "All the whales wanted to follow her."

The last night of my second camping trip, I lie in my tent, my upper arms aching, listening to the staccato rain beat against the nylon. I set my tent up in the middle of a glade of trees, but a few drops of rain still get through. Phil, the friendliest of the engineers, came over to tell me that while I might be all *I am woman, hear me roar*, I had put my tent fly on incorrectly. He also brought word, from the guides, that we'd break camp early in hopes of catching a tailwind back to Smallpox Bay.

I was on the last pages of *Moby-Dick*: "Oh, lonely death on lonely life!" But it was, in the failing light, hard to see the small print. The first morning of the camping trip I'd over-slept and in my rush for the van forgot many of the things I needed. I forgot my flashlight, the small hand-held one, as well as the light attached to the headband that I'd used the year before to go to the outhouse at night. I did not have my cell phone or my warm fleece or my knit cap. I was cold in the tent, and when darkness came I'd be colder still. The trip across the water had been arduous and exhausting; my body ached and I felt old. I had borrowed a plastic bag from one of the guides for my energy-bar wrappers and dirty underwear. I was worried about the plastic bag that I'd put outside between the edge of the tent and the fly. All over the camp, posters warned that food should be tightly secured because the grounds were infested with raccoons. At the bottom of the poster was a photo of a dozen of the animals swarming over a picnic table.

I was worried about the raccoons but my core fears went deeper. As I moved through menopause I often felt death stalking me, just behind my shoulder like a particularly belligerent ghost. Rather than push death away, as I had for years, I was forced to learn to live with her, to accept my body's limitations, accept that the earth's cycle played out not only in the outer world but also inside me. Call it decay or change, I am, like everything else in nature, recyclable. "We learn young," writes the theologian Richard Kearney, "that what disappears as literal comes back again as figural—that is, as sign and symbol, as a second presence in and through absence."

I woke to a sound just to the left of my tent. I lay still under darkness. A darkness in which God had not only shut off the light but also left the building. The rustling stopped, then started again. I felt for *Moby-Dick* and swung the book hard against the side of the tent. The noise stopped. In the quiet I heard an owl's plaintive *whoo whoo*. It was the first time I'd heard the bird in real time, not in a movie or on TV. As the rattling started up and I slapped the book against the thin tent wall, I literally could not see my hands in front of my face.

A woman alone in a pitch-black tent in the middle of the woods can really freak herself out. What if the raccoons were actually bears? What if the engineers and their sons were secret satanists? I alternated between hitting *Moby-Dick* against the nylon and crawling deep inside my sleeping bag, moving my features around in kaleidoscopic expressions of horror.

Of course I flashed continuously, sweat soaking my long johns, matting my bangs to my forehead. I felt as if I was slowly being pulled under, drawn toward the closing vortex. I thought of the revenge of the wild that horror movies played on, that dark force in nature pissed off about clear-cuts and oil spills. In a book I read about the Valdez spill, the author reported finding, on an oil-drenched beach, a black garbage bag filled with dead animals so covered with thick black gunk their species were unidentifiable. I hadn't thought consciously about it before, but animals had every right to take revenge. At this idea I lost my composure completely, flung the book, and then beat my fists against the side of the tent, desperate to frighten off whatever it was that moved in the dark.

◉ ◉ ◉

Is fear always underpinned by death? As I worked on this book, bodies piled up around me. Granny. Colo, the ape from the zoo in Minneapolis. Also loved ones. My eighty-five-year-old friend Miriam. My first husband's mother and his sister, my stepmother and my current husband's mother, my mother-in-law, Gail Hudson. Gail was the first person I'd ever seen die. My husband and I stood next to her hospital bed in New Orleans as blood from a massive stroke moved from the front to the back of her brain. During the first hours, she could have been sleeping, but then her features seemed to sink back in her face and the circles under her eyes turned dark gray. In Gail's last hours, her body struggled to breathe, chest rising and falling mechanically. Finally the breath stopped and her heartbeat slowed, a straightening green line on the monitor above her head. The young resident pressed a stethoscope to her chest for a long while. *She's gone.* Gail's skin took on a delicate lavender color, like the inside of a shell. Her death was what is called peaceful but did nothing to dispel death's mystery. Who was *she* and what was *gone*?

A light came on outside the tent. I recognized the cone of blue as coming from a cell phone. All at once I realized that someone, probably one of the young kayak guides who didn't have a tent, had come to my glade of trees for shelter from the rain. I wasn't going to die—not yet, anyway. My grunts and slaps must have read as extreme restlessness rather than terror. I heard again the rain on the fly and the human just beyond my tent, having finally arranged his air mattress and sleeping bag, give a long, contented sigh.

● ● ●

When I started this book, I assumed we'd soon have our first female post-reproductive, pod-leader president. A killer whale matriarch in the White House. This did not come to pass. What happened instead was a feminist revolution. When I look back on the previous years I can see the swells. From the window of my office at Columbia University I watched Emma Sulkowicz carrying her mattress, draped in black, to protest how little the school did in response to her date rape. My daughter's all-female band, Wilt, came home from college on weekends to play gigs in Brooklyn. They were indignant that at this point in history, they still had to worry about getting attacked when they walked home at night. The women in my literature class complained that while I had picked an equal number of men and women authors, more of the stories focused on the male experience. Also this book you hold in your hands right now! I wanted to fight back, resist how the culture denigrates and stigmatizes menopausal woman. "The menopausal woman," writes Germaine Greer, "is the prisoner of a stereotype and will not be rescued from it until she has begun to tell her own story."

Every ten years or so, I either go back to therapy or I write a book in order to tell myself again, in a new way, my life story. This current version is death heavy, feminism heavy, whale heavy, but also multilayered, even multigenerational. I'm not only fifty-six but also seven, twelve, twenty-seven, thirty-four, and forty-eight. My story is like a choral piece with many different parts. In fact there are so many separate but connected narratives that I sometimes feel a temporal vertigo—I am all ages and no age at all.

◎ ◎ ◎

"If feminism is anything," writes the philosopher Avital Ronell, "it has to be a rigorous call for justice. As long as it excludes certain people, animals and even plants—it's not delivering on its promise."

I make a poster for the Seaquarium protest in Miami. I buy black poster board and neon pink paper. I cut out pink letters—FREE LOLITA—and glue them to the black paper. I get an image of Lolita the whale online and enlarge it ten times on a Xerox machine. Sitting on my bedroom floor, I glue it below the letters. The poster looks wrong, empty. Something is missing. It takes me a few days to realize my poster needs another image, a photo of that other Lolita, the girl held captive inside Nabokov's novel. Even if it's only metaphorical, I can make an alliance with her. On the web, I find a photo of the actress Sue Lyon, who played Lolita in the Kubrick film. I glue-stick her photo beside her namesake's.

"I am not free," wrote Audre Lorde, "while any woman is unfree, even when their shackles are very different from my own."

It's already hot the Saturday in mid-April 2018 when I stand again with protesters outside the Miami Seaquarium. Since September 2017, when Hurricane Irma hit Miami, protests have had more urgency. The Seaquarium sits on a thin strip of land between the city of Miami and Key Biscayne. During Irma, seawater rose up to almost cover the highway. Alejandro Dintiro, who heads the protest along with Mirna Trujillo, tells me Lolita was left alone in her tank during the storm. Wild whales can find places of safety during hurricanes but Lolita was vulnerable. In her small tank she could have been slammed against the concrete wall or hit by missiling debris. If the power went out and the pump stopped, she would be swimming in contaminated water. Lolita would die on display, never able to find out who she was outside the confines of her captivity. "My biggest fear," the former whale trainer Samantha Berg wrote in her blog after Irma, "is that Lolita will die in an illegal tank, just a few yards from the ocean."

After two hours in the hot sun, the adult protesters are wilting, while our youngest member, the twelve-year-old Sara, has taken over the bullhorn. She wears a purple ANIMALS DON'T BELONG IN YOUR STUPID TANKS T-shirt, blue shorts, and tennis shoes. She and her mother, Jessica, came all the way from Delaware to protest. Sara holds up her sign written in black and red marker, 5 ORCAS DIED IN LOLITA'S CAPTURE, and hands out flyers she composed herself: "Ten Reasons Not to Go to the Seaquarium." When I explain that I am working on a book that, in part, is about Lolita, Sara looks at me with what I think is admiration but then realize is recognition. "Me too!" she says.

I feel kinship with Lolita but also with Sara. One of the clear gains of menopause has been a resurgence of my fierce little-girl self. My passion, taken up for a while with the domestic, now lasers out into the wider world. My sense of injustice is sharper and I want to resist. This resistance may itself be an antidote to menopause. "The high anxious but hopeful energy of the time," writes Grace Paley about the 1960s, "the general political atmosphere, and the particular female moment had a lot to do with the fact I can't remember my menopause . . . I've asked some of my age mates, old friends, and they feel pretty much the same way. We were busy. Life was simply heightened by opposition, and hope was essential."

◉ ◉ ◉

Hope is essential. The wild matriarchs have given me hope. No one calls the female whales *roadkill* or *dried-up cunts*. No doctor offers hormone therapy or vaginal rejuvenation. In the matriarchy they've created, children stay with their mothers for life, menopausal females move into leadership roles, and the older post-reproductive females train the adolescent males in sexual technique. While the female whales face nearly insurmountable environmental challenges, each year brings more badassery. They demonstrate to me what no human woman could: that it is not menopause itself that is the problem but menopause as it's experienced under patriarchy. Even in her last months Granny was not side-lined but active. Her large and majestic body diving under and then breaching up and out of the water, hanging over the surface. I remember her seaweedy scent and her brown eye, attentive, wary, and wise. The last photo of her taken by drone, just a few days before she went missing, shows Granny curving her body to corral a salmon for L87, a calf whose mother had recently died. Granny's body may have been breaking down. In the photo she looks thin. "At some point," Giles told me, "she must've decided her life was over, and so she did not go up to breathe at the surface." In death J2 fell down deeper into the sea. I think of my mother's death, the back door flung open to meet that final wildness, to let it in.

◉ ◉ ◉

Menopause is situated at the crossroads between the meta-physical and the biological. It is as much a spiritual challenge as it is a physical one. At this crossroads I have felt haunted by my animalistic past. "We must acknowledge . . . ," Charles Darwin wrote in his 1871 book *The Descent of Man*, "that man with all his noble qualities . . . still bears in his bodily frame the undesirable stamp of his lowly origins." Lowly or not, animals are the main way we know ourselves. The first symbols were animal; the first paintings were of ani-mals. The first metaphors were animal; we judged our speed and fierceness by them. The first religions had animals at their center. "When we speak of the human animal's spontaneous interchanges with the animal landscape," writes the philosopher David Abrams, "we acknowledge a felt relation to the mysterious that was active long before any formal or priestly religion."

"The animal opens before me a depth," writes Georges Bataille, "that attracts me and is familiar to me. In a sense, I know this depth: it is my own. It is also . . . precisely that which is unfathomable to me." I see now that those moments I used to think of as transcendent in a religious sense, when the natural world and its creatures seemed to glow with an inner light, are actually glimpses into my lost animal consciousness.

I don't want to romanticize animals. I know I can't become one of them. But I can stand with them. "The ideal state of human among animals," writes the religion professor Wendy Doniger, "is not one in which wild animals become tame . . . It is a state in which a human becomes one of the animals. Or rather, more precisely, a human becomes part of the society of the animals, but usually remains a human."

◎ ◎ ◎

My fertility continues to expand. I may be aging, even decaying a little, but rot, let's not forget, is generative. It helps new things grow. I'll hunt by reading, writing, volunteering, teaching, protesting, mothering, and loving. And I promise, like a good matriarch, to share the food I find.

Sometimes I think how silly, how human, it was to feel I needed an antidote for menopause: it's like trying to cure a rainstorm, a tulip tendril, or nightfall. As a younger woman, I was led by my biology; now I'll let the spirit tug me along. When I wake in the dark, incandescent with heat, I pray not to a deity up in the sky but to the beauty of this world. I pray the body, I pray the lake, I pray the whale.

A Note About the Whales

In the summer of 2018, as I was finishing this book, J35, a whale known as Tahlequah, gave birth to a daughter. The whale calf died, and her mother, in mourning, carried the dead body of the baby around for seventeen days. Onlookers described J35's vigil as "a ritual or ceremony." Ken Balcomb, head of the Center for Whale Research, called the mother's lament "a very tragic tour of grief."

To me, J35's behavior felt like an act of protest as well as sadness. K, L, and J pods have not had a live birth for almost three years. Pollution and noise hurt the whales, but it's starvation that threatens their existence. The whales eat Chinook salmon, a creature that is overfished and whose migration is blocked by the Lower Snake River dams. We can help the whales by encouraging authorities to increase spill so that more young salmon make it through, as well as pushing for the dam's ultimate removal. We can help the Southern Residents on a daily basis as well by not wasting water or electricity, by biking and carpooling, by recycling, by buying local and organic, by not using household toxins and lawn pesticides. We can also donate to places that support the whales. Places like Wild Orca, www.wildorca.org, and the Center for Whale Research, www.whaleresearch.com.

Maybe L77, a mother that gave birth to a calf in January 2019, will be more fortunate than J35. The calf, nicknamed Lucky, has been seen swimming by its mother's side in the Salish Sea. It's encouraging to see a live calf, though it's the dead one that continues to haunt me. It's one thing to connect to a grieving mother's pain and another to make the changes necessary to help her.

Notes

1. Night on Fire

4 *"About a minute before"*: I interviewed a diverse group of over a hundred women. Interviews were conducted over e-mail, by phone, and in person.

9 *With every flash*: Suzanne Moore, "There Won't Be Blood," *New Statesman*, 2015.

11 *"My feelings seemed"*: Charles Finney, *The Autobiography of Charles G. Finney: The Life Story of America's Greatest Evangelist—in His Own Words* (Bethany House Publishers, 2006).

13 *get back there*: Germaine Greer, *The Change* (Ballantine Books, 1993). While I consider Greer's book to be the best feminist text on menopause, I do not agree with her negation of trans women. Trans women are women. Period.

15 *permeated with alienation*: Joseph F. Brown, "Hulk Smashed! The Rhetoric of Alcoholism in Television's *Incredible Hulk*," *Journal of Popular Culture*, 2011.

19 *estrogen is not the only trigger*: Naomi E. Rance, "Modulation of Body Temperature and LH Secretion by Hypothalamic KNDy Neurons: A Novel Hypothesis on the Mechanism of Hot Flushes," *Frontiers of Neuroendocrinology*, 2013.

2. Free Lolita

22 *killer whales also go through menopause*: Darren P. Croft and Emma A. Foster, "Ecological Knowledge, Leadership, and the Evolution of Menopause in Killer Whales," *Current Biology*, 2015.

23 *only survivor of the Puget Sound capture*: Sandra Pollard, *Puget Sound Whales for Sale: The Fight to End Orca Hunting* (The History Press, 2014), p. 99.

26 *archival footage*: Wolfson Archives, Miami Dade College, Miami, Florida. Thanks to the archivist Lou Kramer.

27 *"I desperately wanted"*: Charles Foster, *Being a Beast* (Picador, 2016), page 10.

34 *"Today I sometimes struggle"*: Jaycee Dugard, *A Stolen Life* (Simon & Schuster, 2011), p. 22.

34 *U.S. Department of Agriculture has finally acknowledged*: Jonathan Kendall, "Lolita's Miami Seaquarium Tank Doesn't Meet Federal Standards," *Miami Times*, March 21, 2016.

3. The Animals

37 *"Something is sent to"*: Edward Tilt, *The Change of Life in Health and Disease* (Lindsay & Blakiston, 1857).

38 *"animal birthday"*: Ernest Becker, *The Denial of Death* (Simon & Schuster, 1973), p. 214.

40 *"I think of my body"*: Carmen Maria Machado, "Unruly, Adjective," *Medium*, 2017.

41 *They are skillful listeners*: Phyllis Lee, "The Reproductive Advantages of a Long Life: Longevity and Senescence in Wild African Elephants," *Behavior Ecology and Sociobiology*, 2016.

41 *matriarchs also distinguish*: Karen Mccomb, *PNAS*, 2014.

44 *"A lot of people ask"*: Sue W. Margulis and Sylvia Atsalis, "Sexual and Hormonal Cycles in Geriatric *Gorilla gorilla gorilla*," *International Journal of Primatology*, 2006.

52 *"There is every indication"*: Georges Bataille, *Theory of Religion* (Zone Books, 1992), p. 35.

4. Mind at the End of Its Tether

57 *While examining a new fifty-one-year-old patient*: Robert A. Wilson, *Feminine Forever* (Pocket Books, 1966) pp. 38–42.

58 *Aristotle thought*: Louise Foxcroft, *Hot Flushes, Cold Science* (Granta Books, 2009). Reading this helped me learn about the earliest history of menopause and how it was misunderstood.

70 *brain is 25 percent different*: Louann Brizendine, *The Female Brain* (Harmony Books, 2006), p. 3.

71 *"I move this body around"*: Samantha Irby, "Hysterical!," *Medium*, 2017.

73 *study in which*: Julie A. Dumas, "Increased Working Memory–Related Brain Activity in Middle-Aged Women with Cognitive Complaints," *Neurobiology of Aging*, 2012.

5. Demigirl in Kemmering

79 *"We must conclude"*: Sigmund Freud, *Lectures on Psycho-Analysis*, 1933.

80 *"hot sexy number"*: Virginie Despentes, *King Kong Theory* (Feminist Press, 2010), p. 8.

85 *"It is fundamental not to"*: Paul B. Preciado, *Testo Junkie* (Feminist Press, 2013), p. 397.

86 *"jumping through a bunch of hoops"*: Juliet Jacques, *Trans: A Memoir* (Verso, 2015), p. 294.

87 *"an ungendering, an unraveling"*: Julia Serano, *Whipping Girl* (Seal Press, 2007), p. 19.

87 *"a unique intensive fire"*: Max Wolf Valerio, *The Testosterone Files* (Seal Press, 2006), p. 9.

6. Lessons in Demonology

98 *how uncomfortable the culture*: Laura J. Petracek, *The Anger Workbook for Women* (New Harbinger, 2004), p. 2.

101 *"If a patient was standing"*: Rick Paulas, "The Neuroscience of Ghosts," *Pacific Standard*, 2016.

102 *often make better ghosts*: Andi Zeisler, "The Feminist Power of Female Ghosts," *Bitch Media*, 2017.

102 *Bloody Mary*: Alan Dundes, "Bloody Mary in the Mirror: A Ritual of Pre-Pubescent Anxiety," *Western Folk Lore* 52, no. 2–3 (1998).

104 *Women could be accused of witchcraft*: These details were collected from a number of sources, among them *The Penguin Book of Witches*, edited by Katherine Howe; *The Witches*, by Stacy Schiff; *The Witch*, by Ronald Hutton; *Witchcraft and the Limits of Interpretation*, by David D. Hall; and *The Devil in the Shape of a Woman*, by Carol F. Karlsen.

109 *One husband told a researcher*: Sue Brayne, *Sex, Meaning and the Menopause* (Continuum, 2011), p. 103.

110 *whatever-you-want-honey hormone*: Julie Holland, *Moody Bitches* (Penguin Press, 2015), p. 39.

7. The Old Monkey

126 *"First there was the shock"*: Ann Mankowitz, *Change of Life* (Inner City Books, 1984), p. 36.

127 *One woman, when she drew a blueprint*: Wendy Maltz and Suzie Boss, *Private Thoughts: Exploring the Power of Women's Sexual Fantasies* (New World Library, 2001), p. 187.

132 *"yet the more we learn"*: Lisa M. Diamond, *Sexual Fluidity* (Harvard University Press, 2008), p. 140.

135 *"Apollo could not enter"*: Elizabeth Abbott, *The History of Celibacy* (Da Capo Press, 1999), p. 37.

137 *half dozen men*: I interviewed men, asking them questions about their own aging bodies and their relationships with their menopausal wives.

140 *seed buried inside*: Barbara G. Walker, *The Crone* (Harper San Francisco, 1985), p. 29.

8. Nocturnal Hunter

148 *"Mama, Mama?"*: Toni Morrison, *Jazz* (Vintage International, 1992), p. 110.

148 *"What does one discover"*: Elena Ferrante, *Frantumaglia* (Europa Editions, 2016), p. 219.

155 "That is the moment": Eve Kosofsky Sedgwick, *Touching Feeling* (Duke University Press, 2003), p. 36.

158 *"is straightforwardly connected"*: Bernard Williams, *Shame and Necessity* (University of California Press, 1993), p. 79.

9. Hole in My Heart

163 *"The vagina is valued"*: Luce Irigaray, *The Sex Which Is Not One* (Cornell University Press, 1985), p. 23.

165 *Even legally the vagina*: Alan Hyde, "The Legal Vagina," *Bodies of Law* (Princeton University Press, 1997).

171 *"I was a body"*: Roxane Gay, *Hunger* (HarperCollins, 2017), p. 10.

173 *"Who is the real subject"*: Anne Carson, *Eros the Bittersweet* (Dalkey Archive Press, 1998), p. 30.

174 *"Our woman with an open pussy"*: Francis Naumann, *The Recurrent, Haunting Ghost: Essays on the Art, Life and Legacy of Marcel Duchamp* (Ready Made Press, 2012).

177 *"There was strength"*: June Arnold, *Sister Gin* (Daughters Inc., 1975), p. 126.

178 *"I'm not dead"*: Kathy Acker, "In Memoriam to Identity," by way of Douglas A. Martin's terrific *Acker* (Nightboat Books, 2017), p. 222.

10. The Whale Wins

186 *"Two seconds went by"*: Erich Hoyt, *Orca: The Whale Called Killer* (Camden House, 1981), p. 54.

187 *"There are so many females"*: Alexander Morton, *Listening to Whales* (Ballantine Books, 2002), p. 139.

191 *orca-gasm*: Tema Milstein's articles helped me understand the experience of whale watching and seeing a whale up close: "Transcorporeal Tourism: Whales, Fetuses and the Rupturing and Reinscribing of Cultural Constraints," *Environmental Communication*, 2012; "When Whales Speak for Themselves: Communication

as a Mediating Force in Wildlife Tourism," *Environmental Communication*, 2008; and "The Performer Metaphor: Mother Nature Never Gives the Same Show Twice," *Environmental Communication*, 2016.

193 *"impossible"*: Jean-Luc Marion, "The Death of the Death of God," *Reimagining the Sacred* (Columbia University Press, 2016), p. 192.

197 *expander of the grandmother hypothesis*: K. Hawkes, J. F. O'Connell, and N. G. Blurton Jones, "Hardworking Hadza Grandmothers," *Comparative Socioecology*, edited by V. Standen and R. A. Foley (Basil Blackwell, 1989); "Grandmothering, Menopause, and the Evolution of Human Life Histories," *Proceedings of the National Academy*, 1998; "Grandmothers and the Evolution of Human Longevity: A Review of Findings and a Future Direction," *Evolutionary Anthropology*, 2013.

11. Home Waters

210 *In a book I read about the Valdez spill*: Eva Saulitis, *Into Great Silence* (Beacon Press, 2013), p. 63.

213 *"If feminism is anything"*: Avital Ronell, *Angry Women* (RE/Search, 1991), p. 140.

213 *"I am not free"*: Audre Lorde, "Uses of Anger," *Sister Outsider* (Crossing Press, 1984), p. 132.

216 *"When we speak of the human animal's"*: David Abrams, *Becoming Animal* (Vintage Books, 2011), p. 277.

217 *"The ideal state of human"*: Wendy Doniger, *The Lives of Animals* (Princeton University Press, 2016), p. 100.

Acknowledgments

This book, more than any of my earlier projects, was a group effort. I interviewed more than a hundred women in person, on the phone, and by e-mail. Their honesty and generosity informed and inspired me. My researchers, Taylor Lannamann, Sarah Levy, and Nicole Starczak, dug up information that made this book better. I am grateful. Lynn Dolnick, Mary Weiss, Sam Kaviar, Dr. Pauline Maki, Dr. Darren Croft, and Dr. Deborah Giles helped me understand animals and human animals.

Thanks to my family and my many friends who supported this book for their enthusiasm and their input: David Steinke, Lauren Steinke, Jonathan Steinke, Nicole LaRosa, Ann Williams, René Steinke, Jill Eisenstadt, Will Blythe, Natalie Standiford, Idra Novey, Elissa Schapell, Rebecca Godfrey, Douglas A. Martin, Bobby Abate, Susan Wheeler, Shelley Jackson, Rob Sheffield, Elizabeth Schmitz, Mitchell Kaplan, Marnie Weber, Bronwyn Keenan, Ben Hudson, Eric Weiner, Jeffrey Greene, Nora O'Connor, Rick Moody, and especially Elizabeth

Mitchell. Biz helped me find the form for this book. A special thanks to my father, the Reverend Paul Steinke: his model of curiosity, empathy, and enthusiasm has been a blueprint for my creative and intellectual life.

Thanks to everyone at FSG: my heroic copy editor, Maureen Klier, and production editor, Susan Goldfarb; also Benjamin Rosenstock and Colin Dickerman. Colin took on this project with a commitment I deeply appreciate. A giant thanks to the great Sarah Crichton, my courageous editor—she is the post-reproductive pod leader I hope to be following for years to come. Kathy Daneman, publicist extraordinaire, helped me get the word out. At the Wylie Agency, to Sarah Chalfant and Jin Auh. Jin has stood by me and my books as a supporter, friend, and confidante for nearly twenty years. Princeton University offered support for research, and the Whiteley Center at the Friday Harbor Labs on San Juan Island gave me a space both to commune with the Southern Resident whales and to write. To my husband, Mike Hudson, who from this book's inception helped me define and clarify my ideas: you supported me with your presence, your care, and your awesome skills as an investigative reporter and an editorial genius. And finally, to my daughter, Abbie Jones, whose fierce millennial feminism continues to challenge and inspire me. In many ways, I wrote this book for you and for your generation.